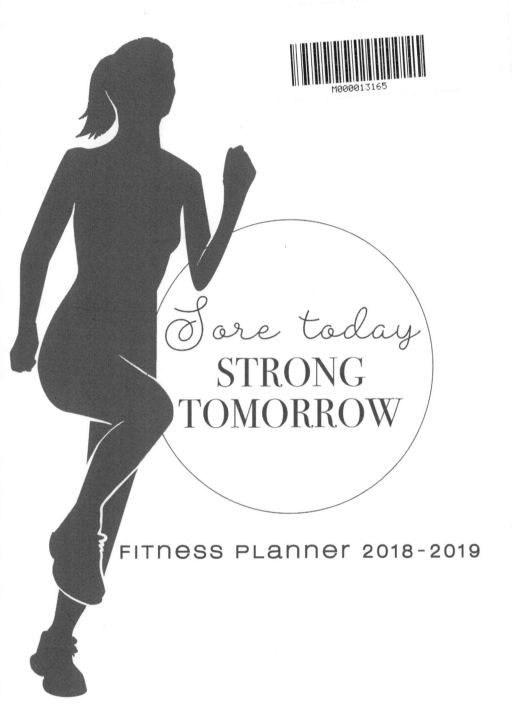

Sore today STRONG TOMORROW

FITNESS PLANNER 2018-2019

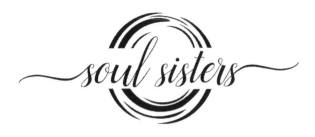

soul sisters

Excuse Me, Gorgeous!
Do you want a chance to win a
LETSCOM Fitness Tracker HR
and take your fitness journey to the next level?!

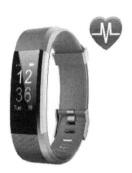

LETSCOM Fitness Tracker HR includes:

Activity Tracker with Heart Rate Monitor Watch, IP67

Waterproof Smart Wristband with Calorie Counter,

Pedometer, and a Sleep Monitor!

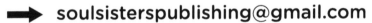

Simply, email us with your feedback about on our new **Sore Today, Strong Tomorrow Fitness Planner** and we will select an entry every other month for this beautiful watch!

Email us at:

➡ soulsisterspublishing@gmail.com ⬅

If you enjoy our products, please leave us a review on Amazon to help support our small business!
After all, you are our INSPIRATION!

With love,
Emma & Anna

 Follow Us on Facebook:
Soul Sisters

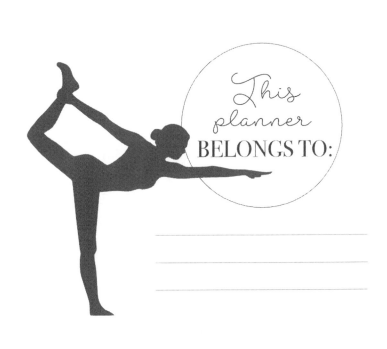

This
planner
BELONGS TO:

_____

_____

_____

CARDIO: Exercise   Duration   Cals.
                                                                  Burned

_____   _____   _____

_____   _____   _____

_____   _____   _____

STRETCH: Cool-down   TIME

_____   _____

_____   _____

_____   _____

Workout
TRACKER

1	2	3	4	5	6	7	8
9	10	11	12	13	14	15	16
17	18	19	20	21	22	23	24
25	26	27	28	29	30	31	

Habits TRACKER

Everyday habits

1		4	
2		5	
3		6	

	1	2	3	4	5	6		1	2	3	4	5	6
1							17						
2							18						
3							19						
4							20						
5							21						
6							22						
7							23						
8							24						
9							25						
10							26						
11							27						
12							28						
13							29						
14							30						
15							31						
16													

Plan
AHEAD

Date: _____ _____ _____ TO _____ _____ _____

	Current	Goal
Weight:		
Body fat %:		
Energy Level:		
Other:		

This week's plan

Work out schedule: **S   M   T   W   T   F   S**

Nutrition: _____

_____

_____

Goals: _____

_____

_____

Reward

_____

_____

_____

_____

_____

Notes

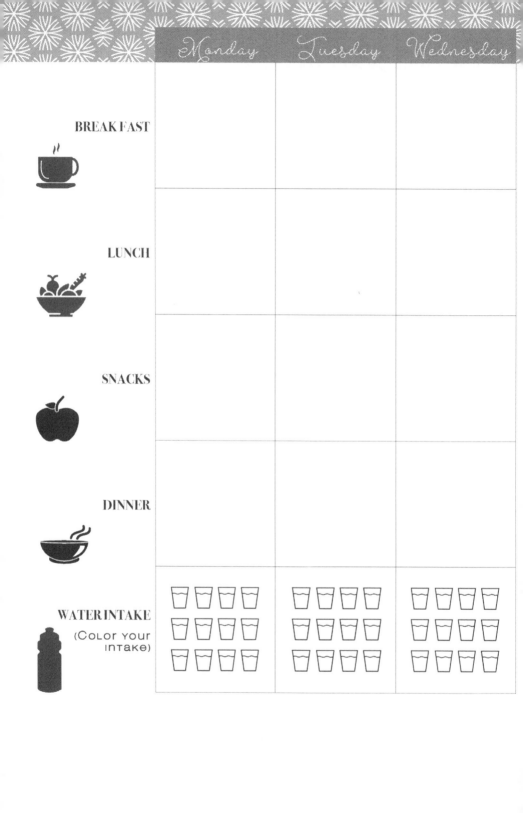

	Monday	Tuesday	Wednesday
BREAKFAST			
LUNCH			
SNACKS			
DINNER			
WATER INTAKE (Color your intake)			

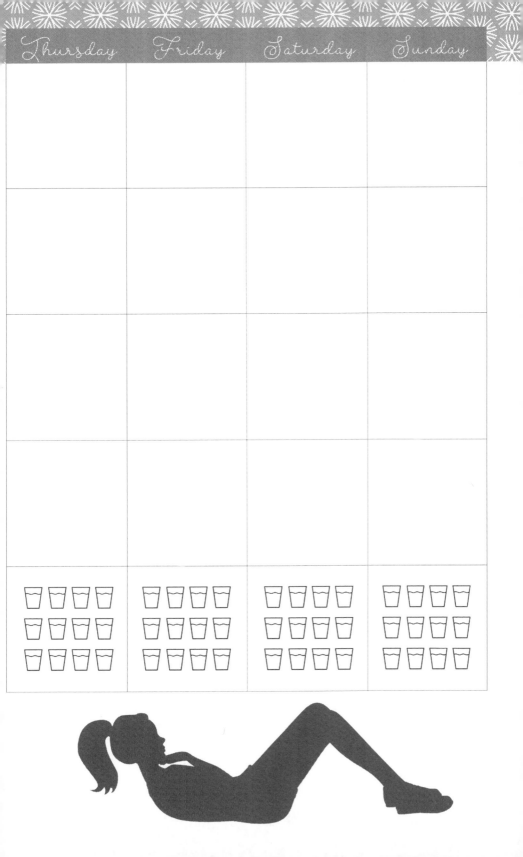

Plan AHEAD

Date: _____ _____ _____   to _____ _____ _____

	Current	Goal
Weight:		
Body fat %:		
Energy Level:		
Other:		

This week's plan

Work out schedule: S   M   T   W   T   F   S

Nutrition: _____
_____
_____

Goals: _____
_____
_____

Reward

_____
_____
_____
_____
_____

Notes

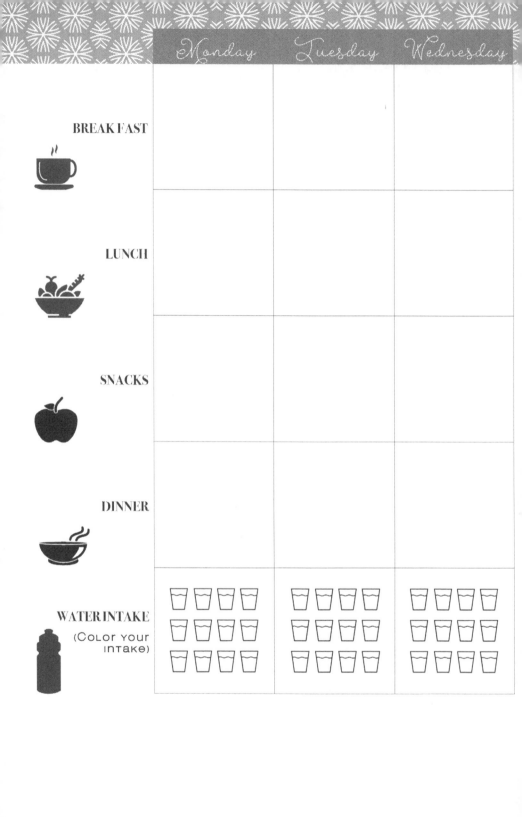

	Monday	Tuesday	Wednesday
BREAK FAST			
LUNCH			
SNACKS			
DINNER			
WATER INTAKE (Color your intake)			

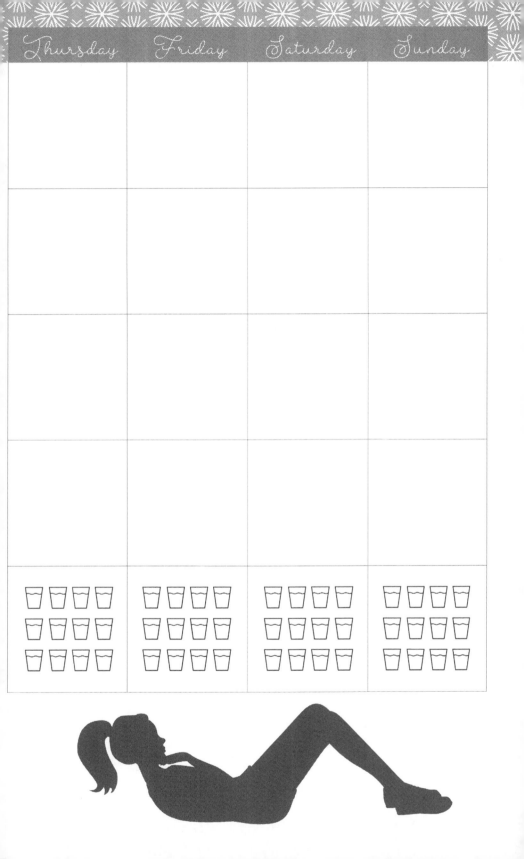

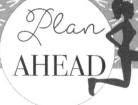

Plan AHEAD

Date: _____ _____ _____   to   _____ _____ _____

	Current	Goal
Weight:		
Body fat %:		
Energy Level:		
Other:		

This week's plan

Work out schedule: **S   M   T   W   T   F   S**

Nutrition:
_____
_____
_____

Goals:
_____
_____
_____

Reward

_____
_____
_____
_____
_____

Notes

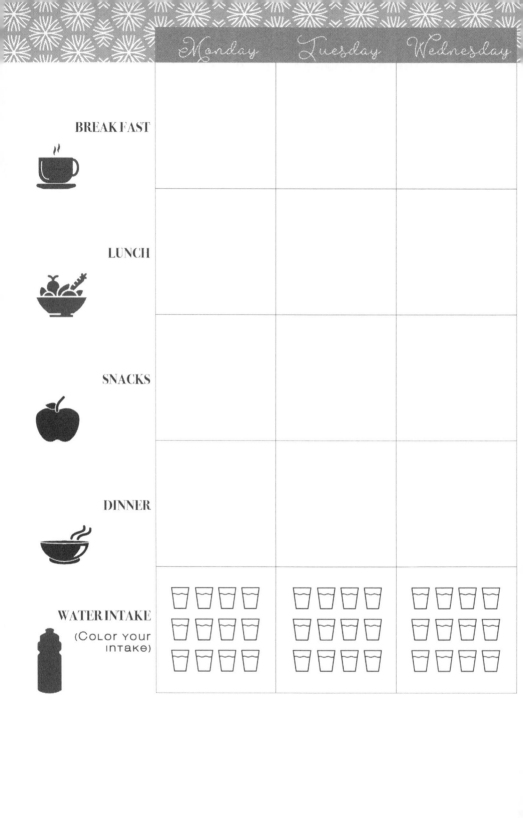

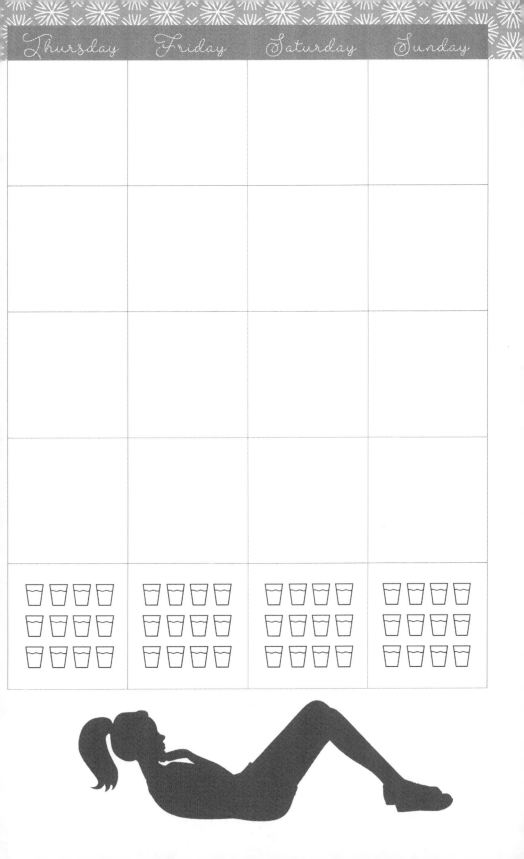

Plan
AHEAD

Date: _____ TO _____

	Current	Goal
Weight:		
Body fat %:		
Energy Level:		
Other:		

This week's plan

Work out schedule: **S   M   T   W   T   F   S**

Nutrition:
_____
_____
_____

Goals:
_____
_____
_____

Reward

_____
_____
_____
_____
_____

Notes

_____
_____
_____
_____
_____
_____
_____
_____
_____
_____
_____
_____
_____
_____
_____
_____
_____
_____
_____
_____
_____
_____

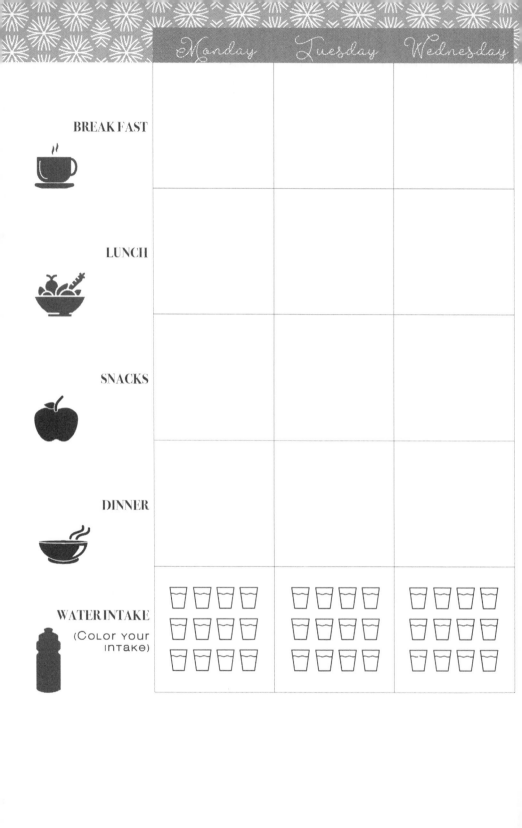

Thursday	Friday	Saturday	Sunday

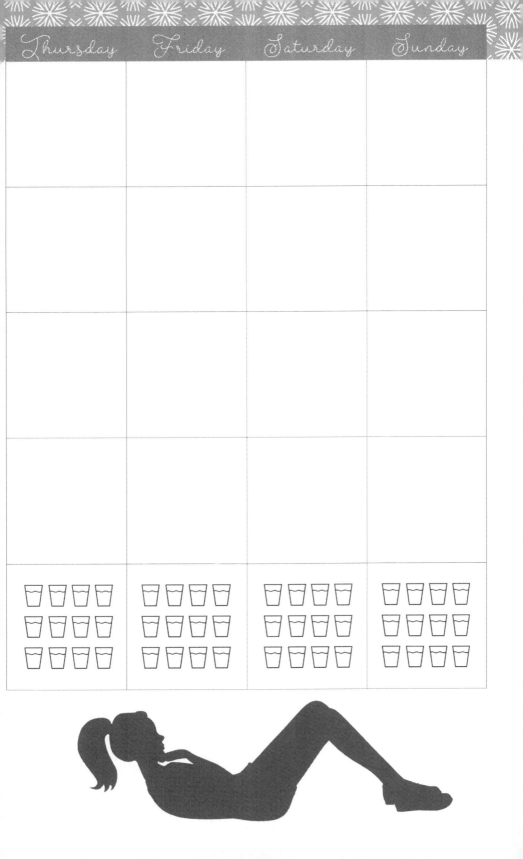

Strength Training

Exercise	Reps.	Sets	Focus

Notes

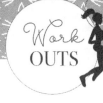

Work
OUTS

CARDIO: Exercise

Duration

Cals.
Burned

_____   _____   _____

_____   _____   _____

_____   _____   _____

STRETCH: Cool-down

TIME

_____   _____

_____   _____

_____   _____

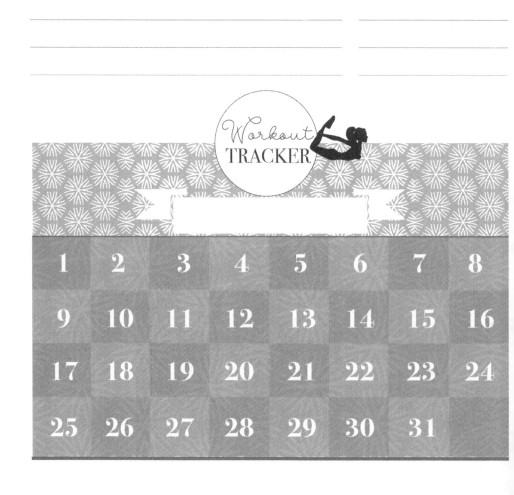

Workout
TRACKER

1	2	3	4	5	6	7	8
9	10	11	12	13	14	15	16
17	18	19	20	21	22	23	24
25	26	27	28	29	30	31	

Everyday habits

1 _____		4 _____
2 _____		5 _____
3 _____		6 _____

	1	2	3	4	5	6		1	2	3	4	5	6
1							17						
2							18						
3							19						
4							20						
5							21						
6							22						
7							23						
8							24						
9							25						
10							26						
11							27						
12							28						
13							29						
14							30						
15							31						
16													

Plan
AHEAD

Date: _____ _____ _____ TO _____ _____

	Current	Goal
Weight:		
Body fat %:		
Energy Level:		
Other:		

This week's plan

Work out schedule: **S   M   T   W   T   F   S**

Nutrition: _____

_____

_____

Goals: _____

_____

_____

Reward

_____

_____

_____

_____

_____

Notes

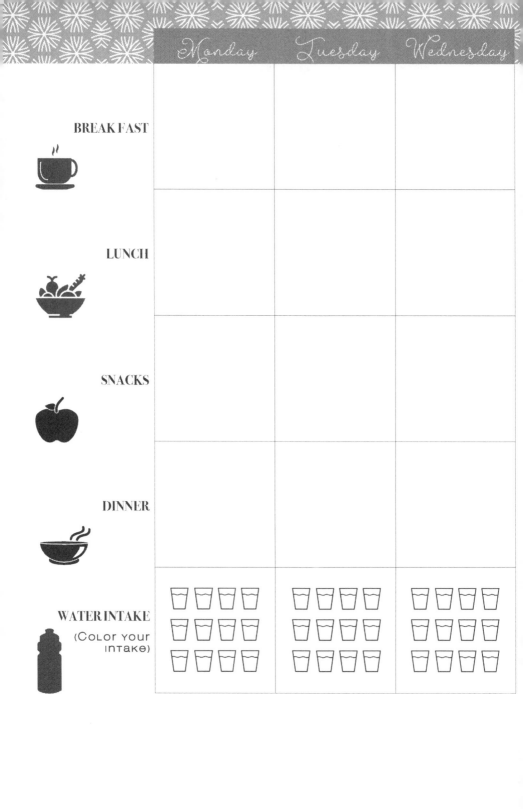

	Monday	Tuesday	Wednesday
BREAK FAST			
LUNCH			
SNACKS			
DINNER			
WATER INTAKE (Color your intake)			

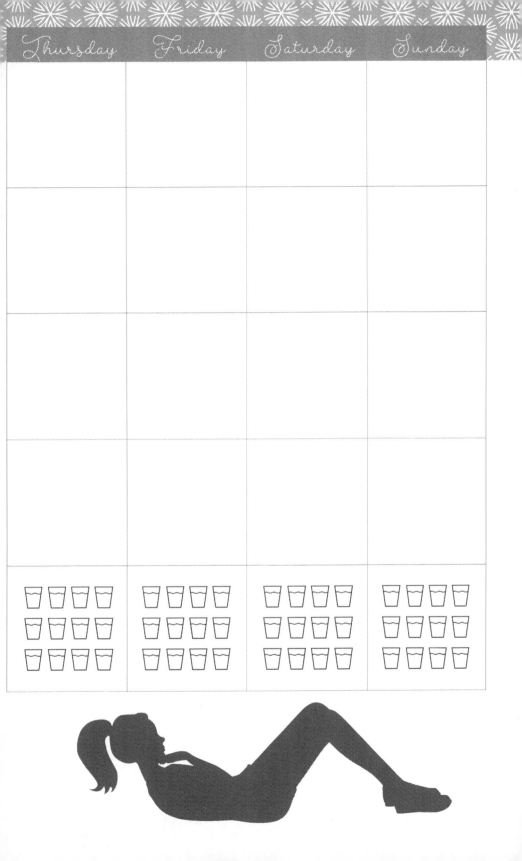

Plan AHEAD

Date: _____ _____ _____   TO _____ _____ _____

	Current	Goal
Weight:		
Body fat %:		
Energy Level:		
Other:		

This week's plan

Work out schedule: **S   M   T   W   T   F   S**

Nutrition:
_____
_____
_____

Goals:
_____
_____
_____

Reward
_____
_____
_____
_____
_____

Notes

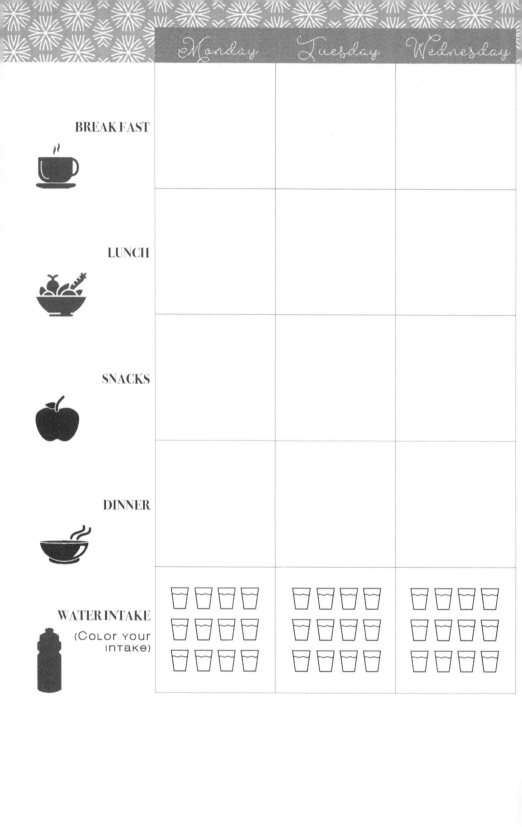

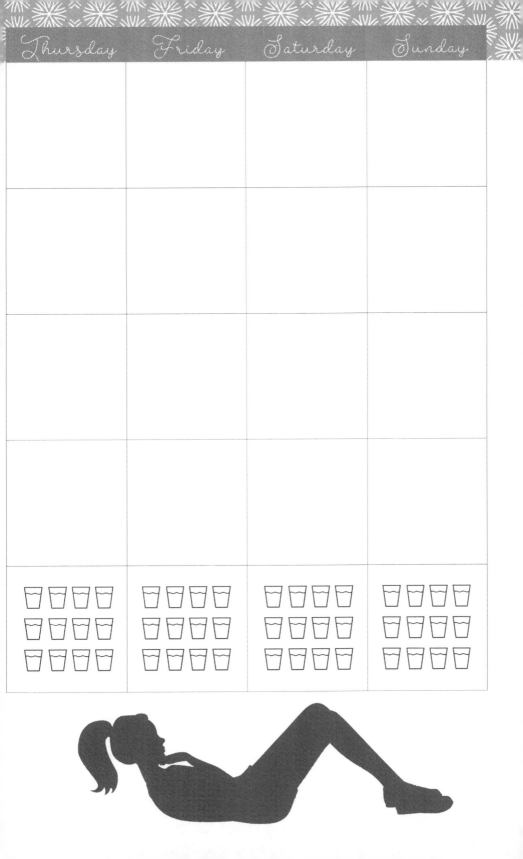

Thursday	Friday	Saturday	Sunday

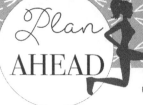

Plan AHEAD

Date: ———— ———— ———— TO ———— ———— ————

	Current	Goal
Weight:		
Body fat %:		
Energy Level:		
Other:		

This week's plan

Work out schedule: **S   M   T   W   T   F   S**

Nutrition:

_____

_____

Goals:

_____

_____

Reward

_____

_____

_____

Notes

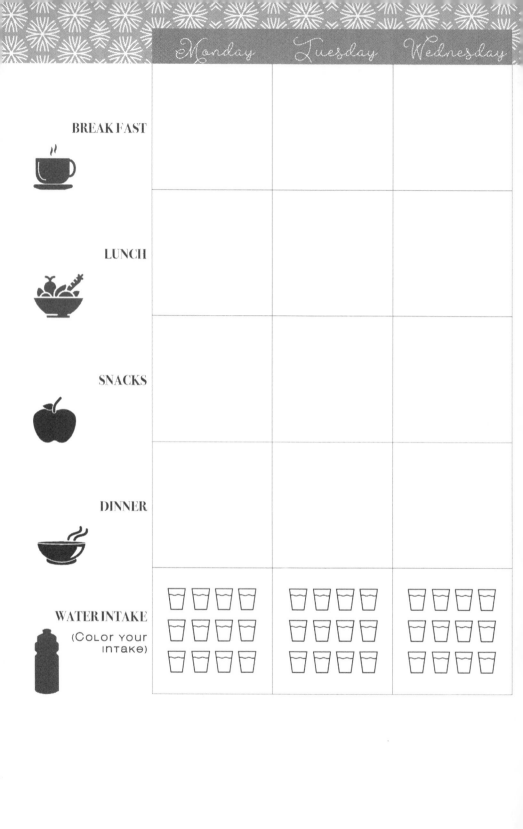

	Monday	Tuesday	Wednesday
BREAK FAST			
LUNCH			
SNACKS			
DINNER			
WATER INTAKE (Color your intake)			

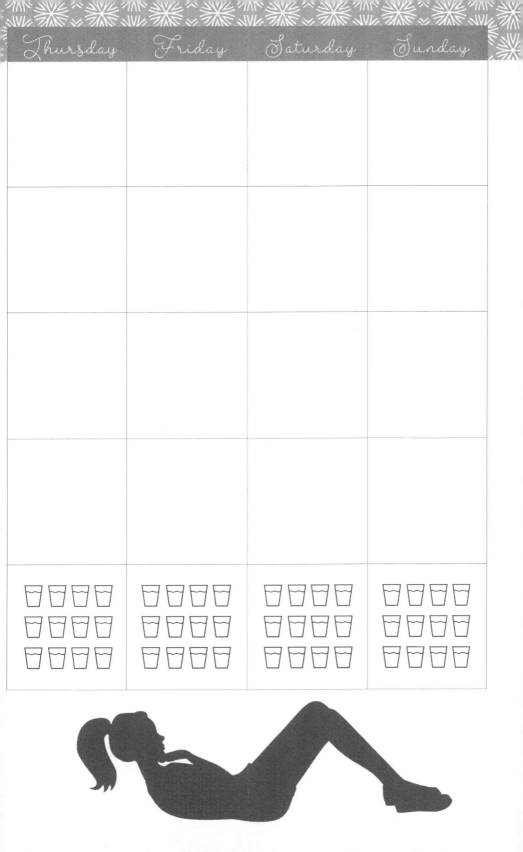

Thursday	Friday	Saturday	Sunday

Plan AHEAD

Date: _____ _____ _____ TO _____ _____ _____

	Current	Goal
Weight:		
Body fat %:		
Energy Level:		
Other:		

This week's plan

Work out schedule: S   M   T   W   T   F   S

Nutrition:
_____
_____

Goals:
_____
_____
_____

Reward

_____
_____
_____
_____
_____

Notes

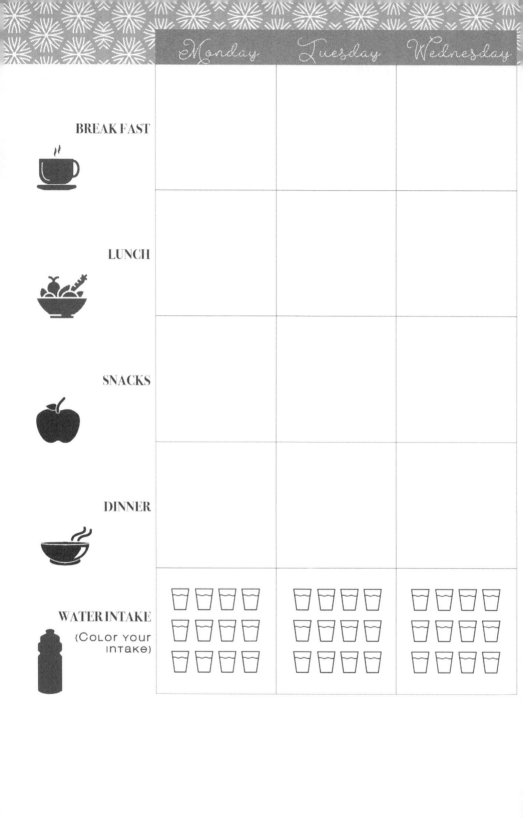

	Monday	Tuesday	Wednesday
BREAKFAST			
LUNCH			
SNACKS			
DINNER			
WATER INTAKE (Color your intake)			

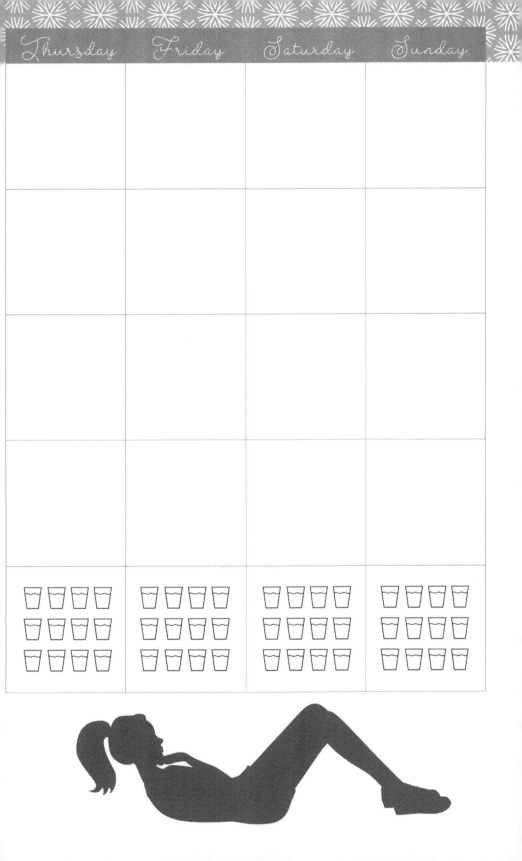

Strength Training

Exercise	Reps.	Sets	Focus

Notes

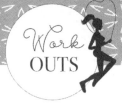

Work
OUTS

CARDIO: Exercise   Duration   Cals. Burned

_____   _____   _____

_____   _____   _____

_____   _____   _____

STRETCH: Cool-down   TIME

_____   _____

_____   _____

_____   _____

Workout
TRACKER

1	2	3	4	5	6	7	8
9	10	11	12	13	14	15	16
17	18	19	20	21	22	23	24
25	26	27	28	29	30	31	

Habits TRACKER

Everyday habits

1 _____   4 _____

2 _____   5 _____

3 _____   6 _____

	1	2	3	4	5	6		1	2	3	4	5	6
1							17						
2							18						
3							19						
4							20						
5							21						
6							22						
7							23						
8							24						
9							25						
10							26						
11							27						
12							28						
13							29						
14							30						
15							31						
16													

Plan AHEAD

Date: _____ _____ _____ TO _____ _____ _____

	Current	Goal
Weight:		
Body fat %:		
Energy Level:		
Other:		

This week's plan

Work out schedule: **S   M   T   W   T   F   S**

Nutrition:
_____
_____
_____

Goals:
_____
_____
_____

Reward
_____
_____
_____
_____
_____

Notes

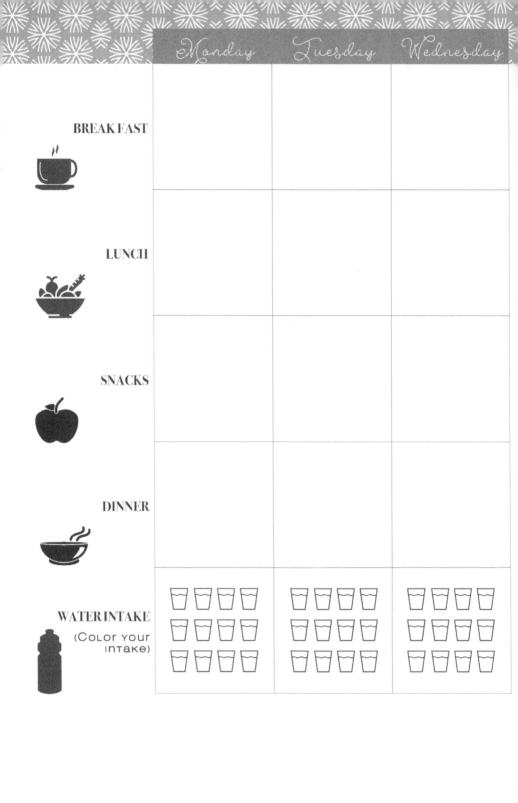

	Monday	Tuesday	Wednesday
BREAKFAST			
LUNCH			
SNACKS			
DINNER			
WATER INTAKE (Color your intake)			

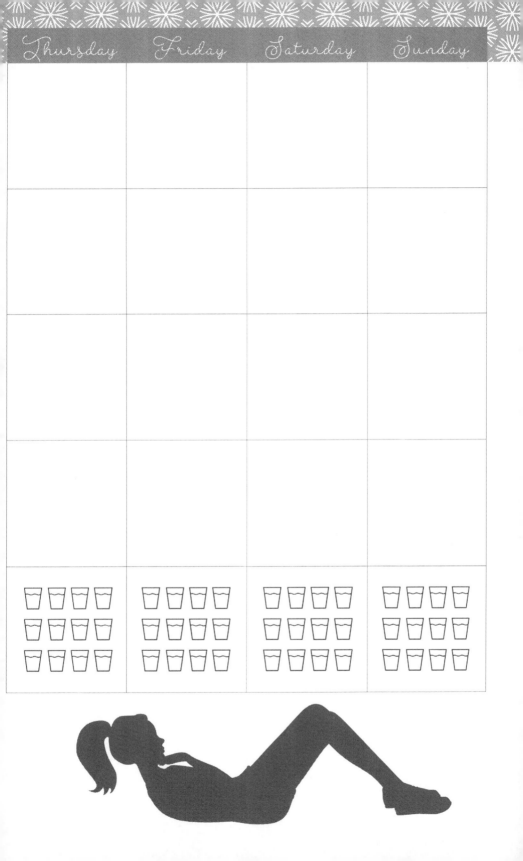

Thursday	Friday	Saturday	Sunday

Plan AHEAD

Date: _____ _____ _____   TO _____ _____ _____

	Current	Goal
Weight:		
Body fat %:		
Energy Level:		
Other:		

This week's plan

Work out schedule: S   M   T   W   T   F   S

Nutrition: _____
_____
_____

Goals: _____
_____
_____

Reward

_____
_____
_____
_____
_____

Notes

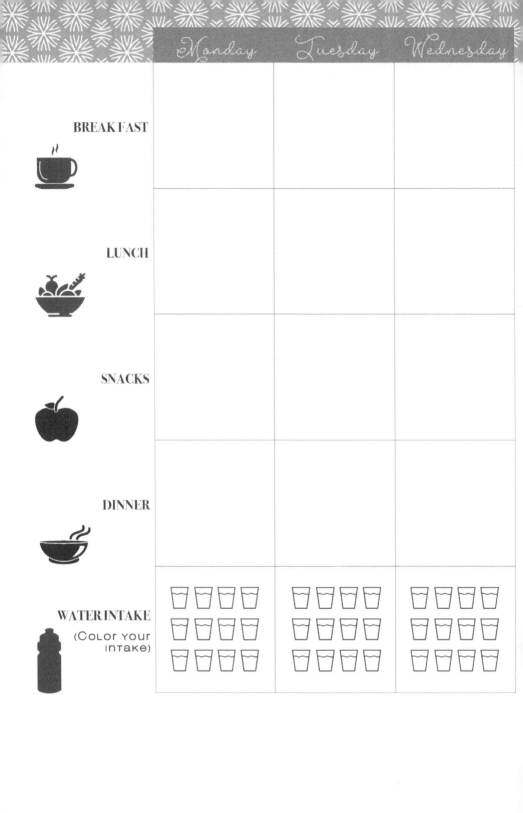

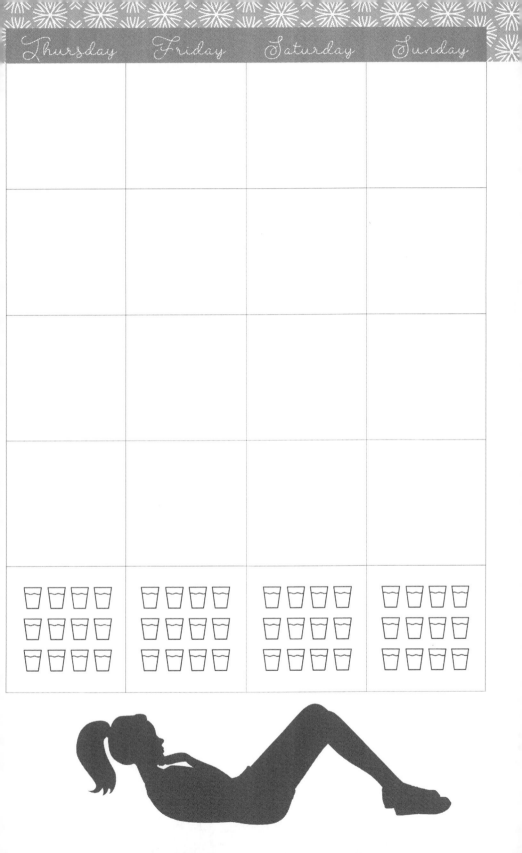

Plan
AHEAD

Date: _____ _____ _____   TO   _____ _____

	Current	Goal
Weight:		
Body fat %:		
Energy Level:		
Other:		

This week's plan

Work out schedule: S   M   T   W   T   F   S

Nutrition:
_____
_____
_____

Goals:
_____
_____
_____

Reward
_____
_____
_____
_____
_____

Notes

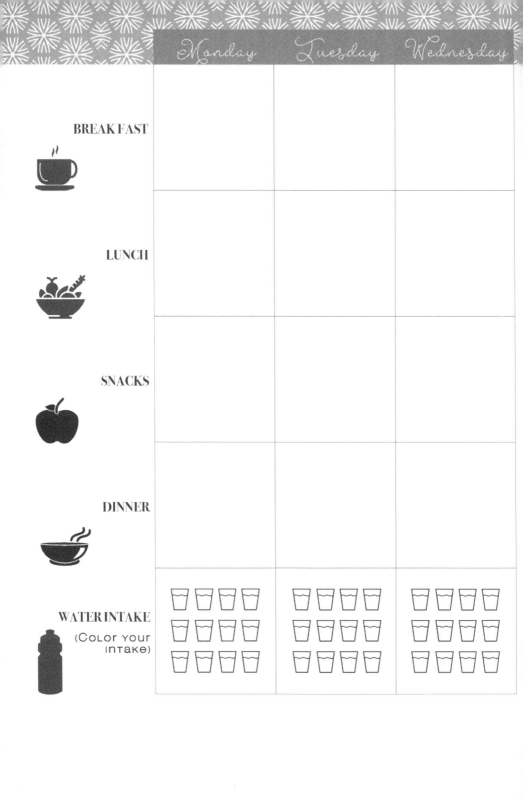

	Monday	Tuesday	Wednesday
BREAKFAST			
LUNCH			
SNACKS			
DINNER			
WATER INTAKE (Color your intake)			

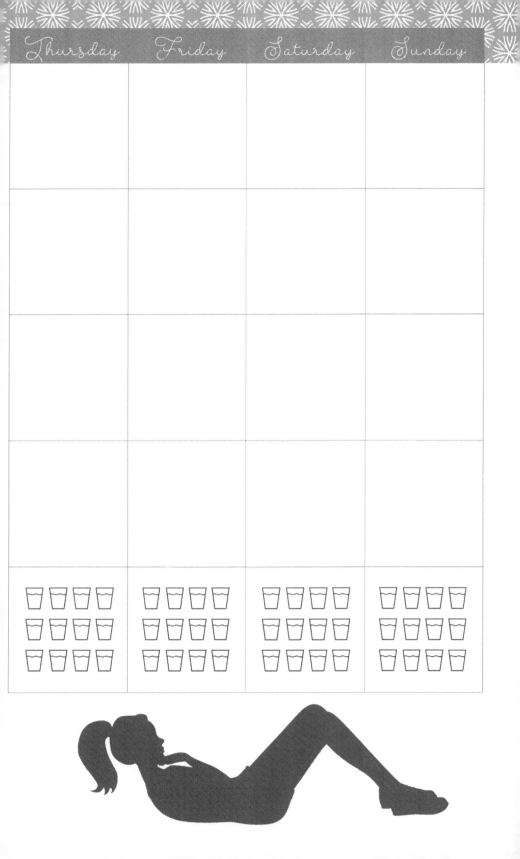

Plan
AHEAD

Date: _____ _____ _____   to _____ _____ _____

	Current	Goal
Weight:		
Body fat %:		
Energy Level:		
Other:		

This week's plan

Work out schedule: **S   M   T   W   T   F   S**

Nutrition: _____

_____

_____

Goals: _____

_____

_____

Reward

_____

_____

_____

_____

_____

Notes

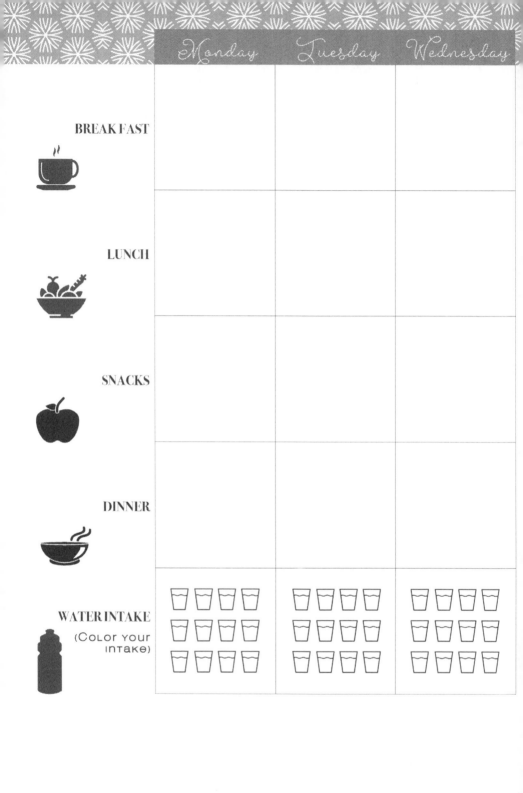

	Monday	Tuesday	Wednesday
BREAKFAST			
LUNCH			
SNACKS			
DINNER			
WATER INTAKE (Color your intake)			

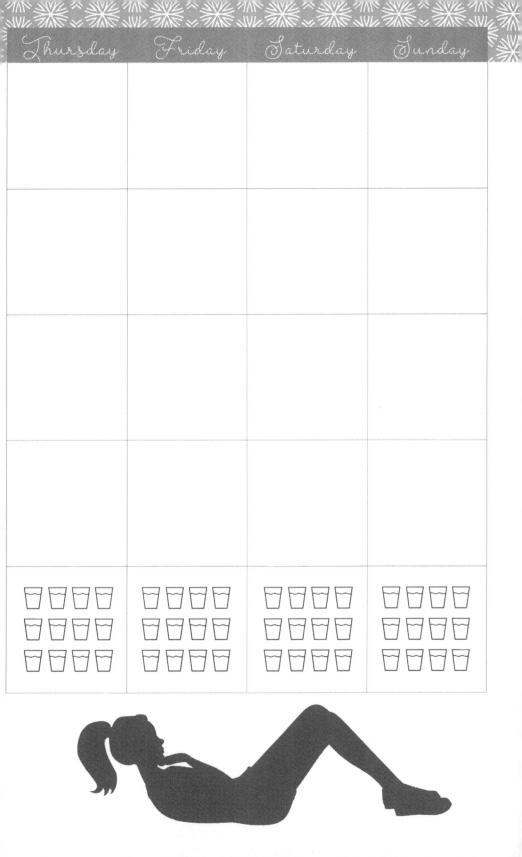

Strength Training

Exercise	Reps.	Sets	Focus

Notes

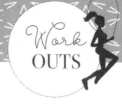

Work
OUTS

CARDIO: Exercise   Duration   Cals. Burned

_____   _____   _____
_____   _____   _____
_____   _____   _____

STRETCH: Cool-down   TIME

_____   _____
_____   _____
_____   _____

Workout
TRACKER

1	2	3	4	5	6	7	8
9	10	11	12	13	14	15	16
17	18	19	20	21	22	23	24
25	26	27	28	29	30	31	

Habits TRACKER

Everyday habits

1	4
2	5
3	6

	1	2	3	4	5	6		1	2	3	4	5	6
1							17						
2							18						
3							19						
4							20						
5							21						
6							22						
7							23						
8							24						
9							25						
10							26						
11							27						
12							28						
13							29						
14							30						
15							31						
16													

Plan
AHEAD

Date: _____ _____ _____ TO _____ _____ _____

	Current	Goal
Weight:		
Body fat %:		
Energy Level:		
Other:		

This week's plan

Work out schedule: **S M T W T F S**

Nutrition:

_____

_____

Goals:

_____

_____

_____

Reward

_____

_____

_____

_____

_____

Notes

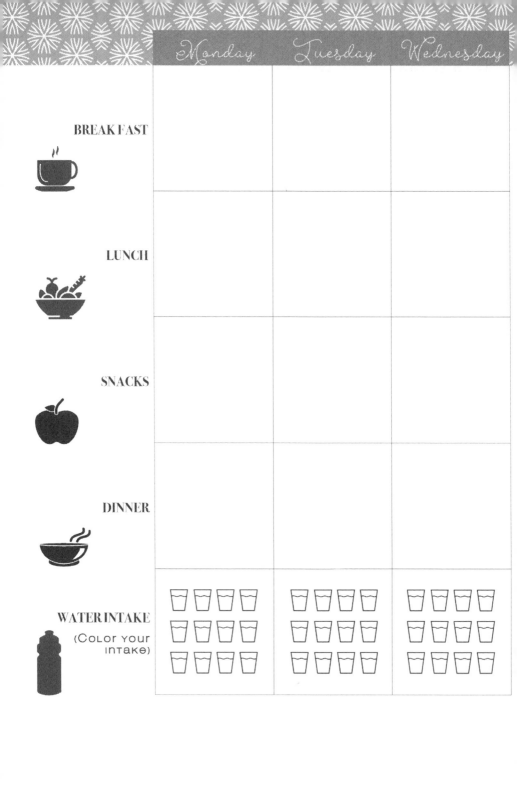

	Monday	Tuesday	Wednesday
BREAKFAST			
LUNCH			
SNACKS			
DINNER			
WATER INTAKE (Color your intake)			

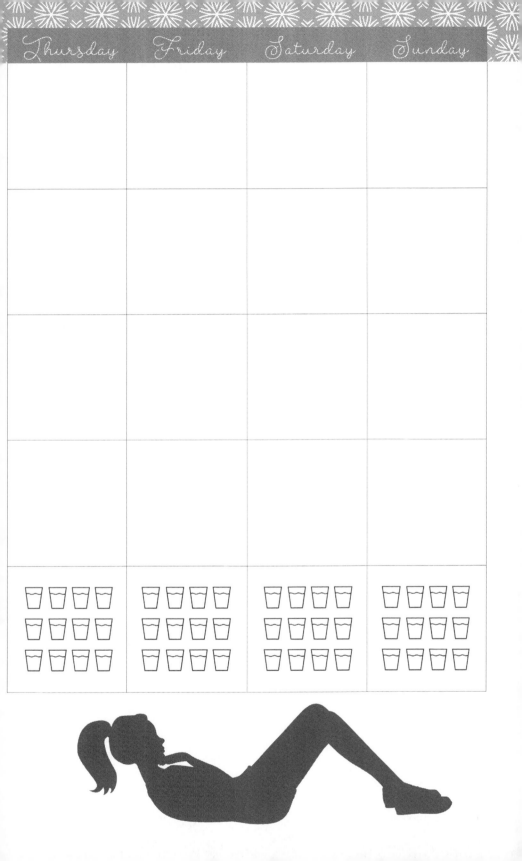

Thursday	Friday	Saturday	Sunday

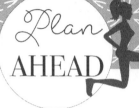

Plan AHEAD

Date: _____ _____ _____ TO _____ _____ _____

	Current	Goal
Weight:		
Body fat %:		
Energy Level:		
Other:		

This week's plan

Work out schedule: S   M   T   W   T   F   S

Nutrition: _____
_____
_____

Goals: _____
_____
_____

Reward

_____
_____
_____
_____

Notes

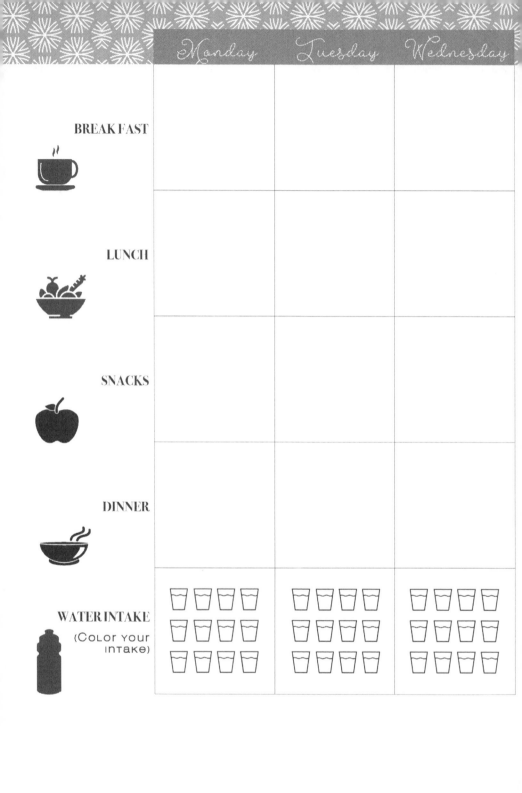

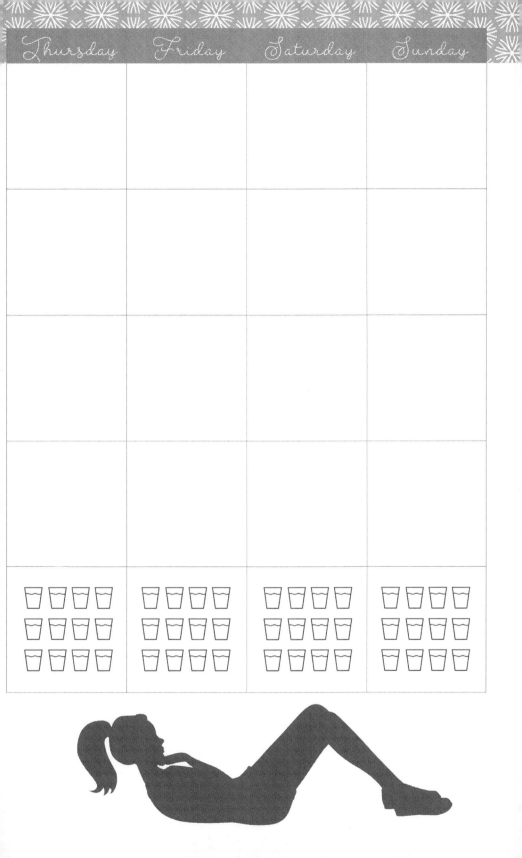

Thursday	Friday	Saturday	Sunday

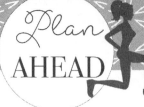

Plan
AHEAD

Date: _____ to _____

	Current	Goal
Weight:		
Body fat %:		
Energy Level:		
Other:		

This week's plan

Work out schedule: **S   M   T   W   T   F   S**

Nutrition: _____

_____

_____

Goals: _____

_____

_____

Reward

_____

_____

_____

_____

_____

Notes

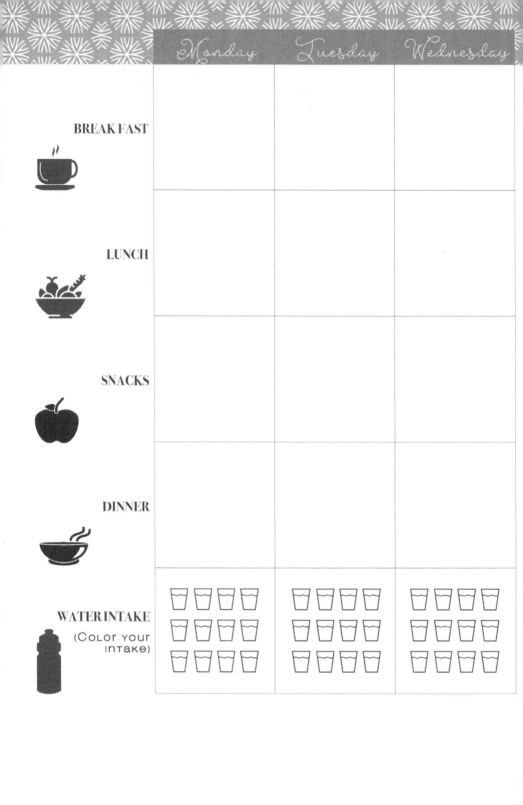

	Monday	Tuesday	Wednesday
BREAKFAST			
LUNCH			
SNACKS			
DINNER			
WATER INTAKE (Color your intake)			

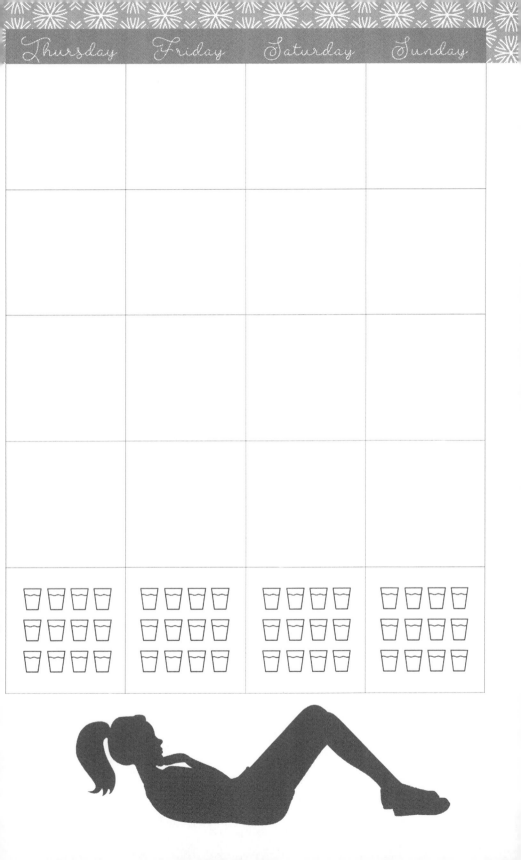

Thursday	Friday	Saturday	Sunday

Plan AHEAD

Date: _____ _____ _____   to   _____ _____ _____

	Current	Goal
Weight:		
Body fat %:		
Energy Level:		
Other:		

This week's plan

Work out schedule: **S**   **M**   **T**   **W**   **T**   **F**   **S**

Nutrition: _____
_____
_____

Goals: _____
_____
_____
_____

Reward

_____
_____
_____
_____
_____

Notes

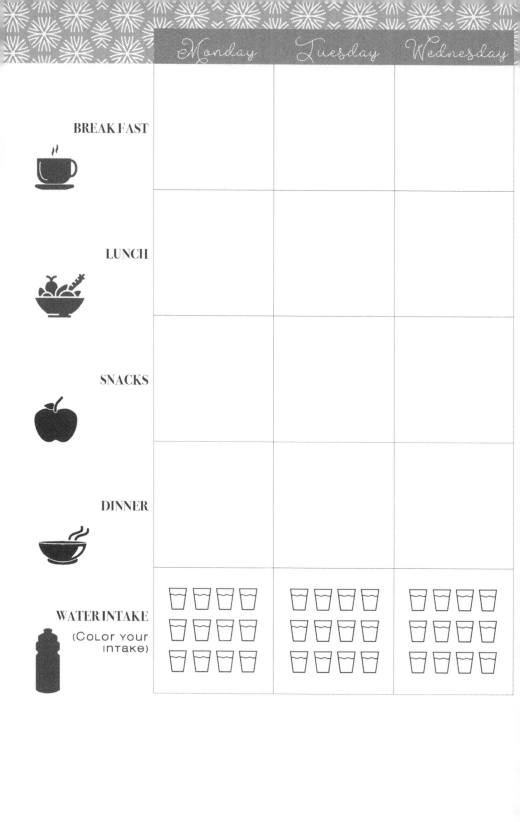

	Monday	Tuesday	Wednesday
BREAKFAST			
LUNCH			
SNACKS			
DINNER			
WATER INTAKE (Color your intake)			

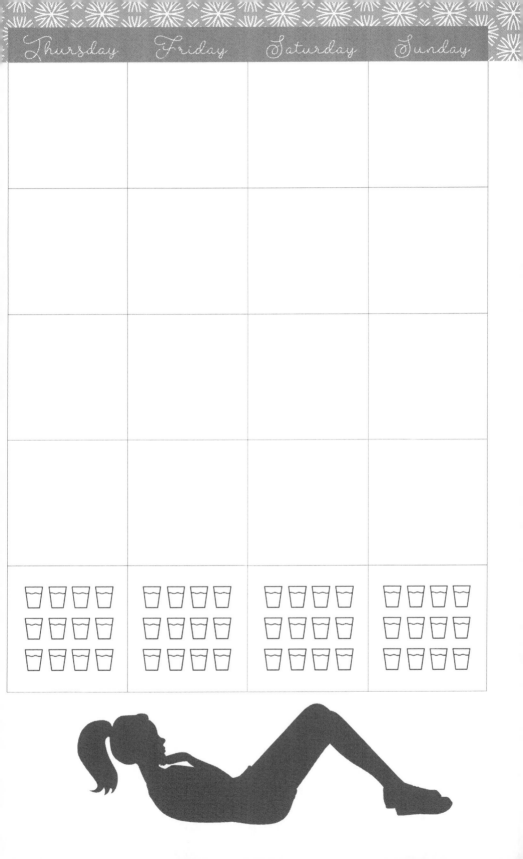

Strength Training

Exercise	Reps.	Sets	Focus

Notes

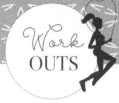

Work
OUTS

CARDIO: Exercise · Duration · · · · Cals. Burned

_____ · · · · · · _____ · · · · · · _____

_____ · · · · · · _____ · · · · · · _____

_____ · · · · · · _____ · · · · · · _____

STRETCH: Cool-down · TIME

_____ · · · · · · _____

_____ · · · · · · _____

_____ · · · · · · _____

Workout
TRACKER

1	2	3	4	5	6	7	8
9	10	11	12	13	14	15	16
17	18	19	20	21	22	23	24
25	26	27	28	29	30	31	

Habits TRACKER

Everyday habits

1 _____   4 _____
2 _____   5 _____
3 _____   6 _____

	1	2	3	4	5	6			1	2	3	4	5	6
1							17							
2							18							
3							19							
4							20							
5							21							
6							22							
7							23							
8							24							
9							25							
10							26							
11							27							
12							28							
13							29							
14							30							
15							31							
16														

Plan
AHEAD

Date: _____ _____ _____ to _____ _____ _____

	Current	Goal
Weight:		
Body fat %:		
Energy Level:		
Other:		

This week's plan

Work out schedule: S M T W T F S

Nutrition: _____
_____
_____

Goals: _____
_____
_____
_____

Reward

_____
_____
_____
_____
_____

Notes

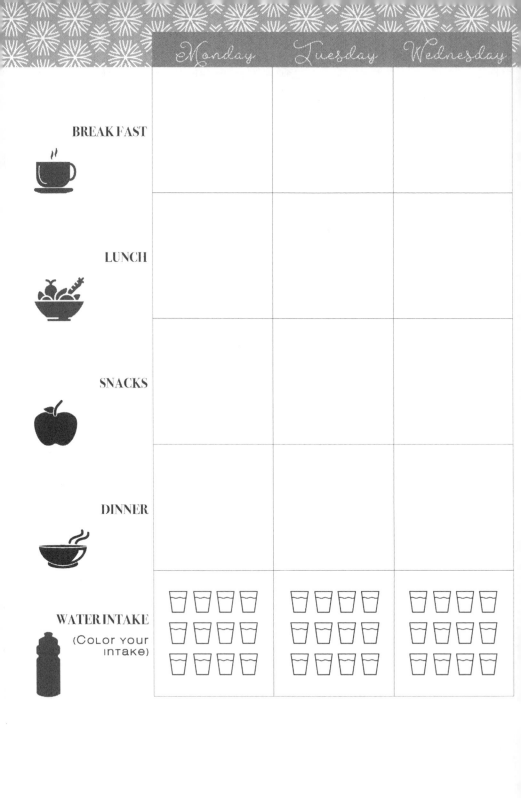

	Monday	Tuesday	Wednesday
BREAK FAST			
LUNCH			
SNACKS			
DINNER			
WATER INTAKE (Color your intake)			

Thursday	Friday	Saturday	Sunday
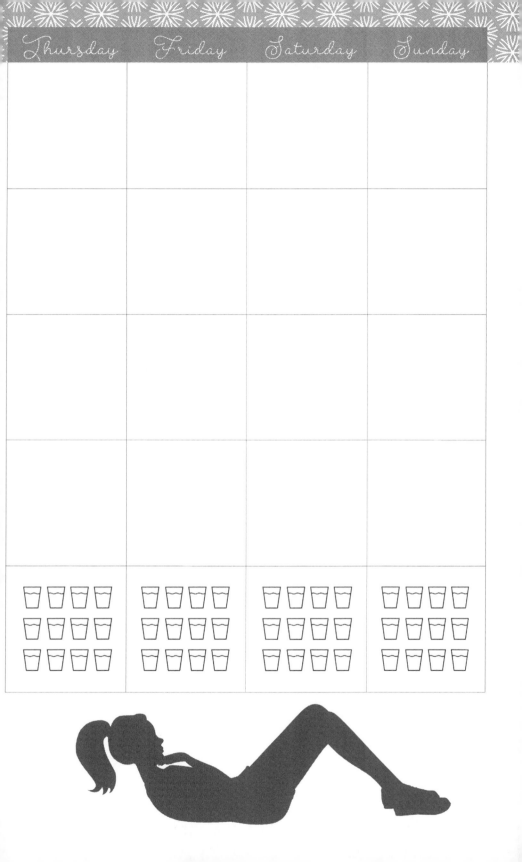

Plan
AHEAD

Date: _____ _____ _____ TO _____ _____ _____

	Current	Goal
Weight:		
Body fat %:		
Energy Level:		
Other:		

This week's plan

Work out schedule: **S   M   T   W   T   F   S**

Nutrition:
_____
_____

Goals:
_____
_____
_____

Reward

_____
_____
_____
_____
_____

Notes

_____
_____
_____
_____
_____
_____
_____
_____
_____
_____
_____
_____
_____
_____
_____
_____
_____
_____
_____
_____
_____

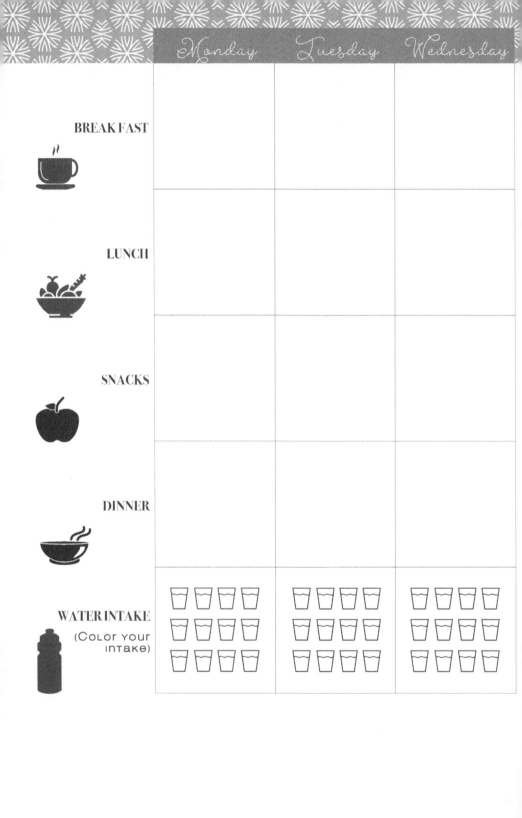

	Monday	Tuesday	Wednesday
BREAKFAST			
LUNCH			
SNACKS			
DINNER			
WATER INTAKE (Color your intake)			

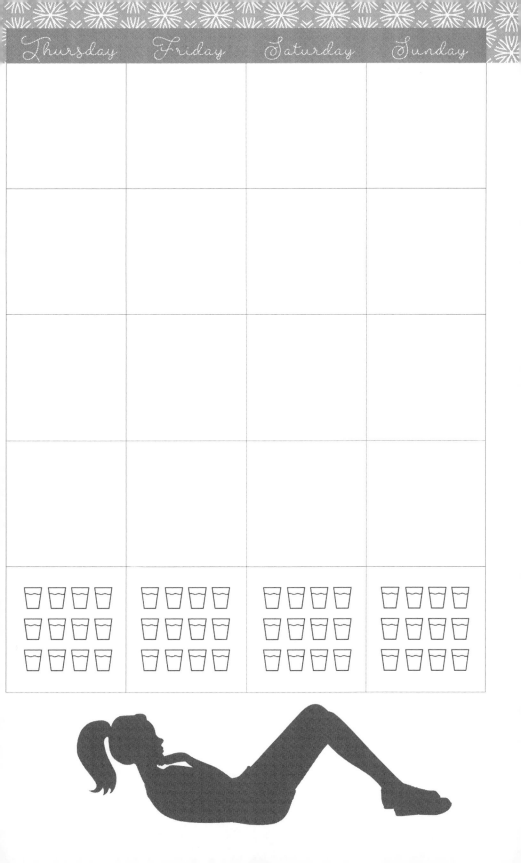

Plan
AHEAD

Date: _____ to _____

	Current	Goal
Weight:		
Body fat %:		
Energy Level:		
Other:		

This week's plan

Work out schedule: **S   M   T   W   T   F   S**

Nutrition: _____

_____

_____

Goals: _____

_____

_____

Reward

_____

_____

_____

_____

_____

Notes

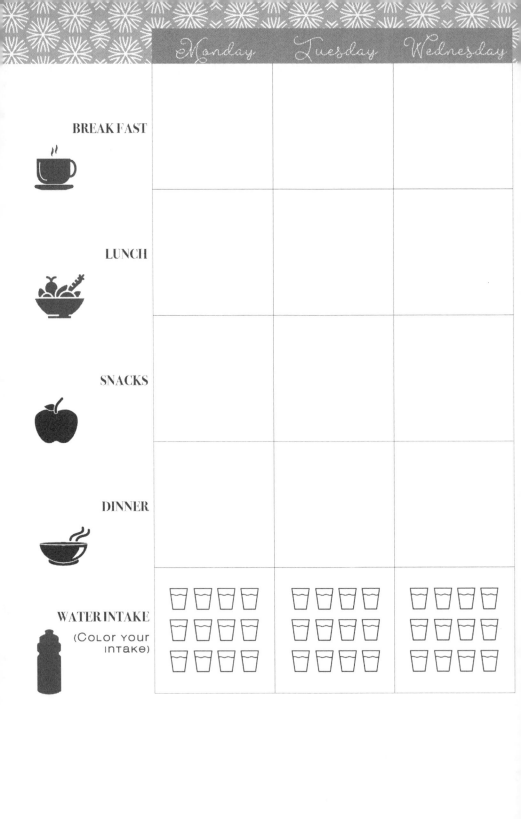

	Monday	Tuesday	Wednesday
BREAKFAST			
LUNCH			
SNACKS			
DINNER			
WATER INTAKE (Color your intake)			

🥛🥛🥛🥛 🥛🥛🥛🥛 🥛🥛🥛🥛	🥛🥛🥛🥛 🥛🥛🥛🥛 🥛🥛🥛🥛	🥛🥛🥛🥛 🥛🥛🥛🥛 🥛🥛🥛🥛	🥛🥛🥛🥛 🥛🥛🥛🥛 🥛🥛🥛🥛

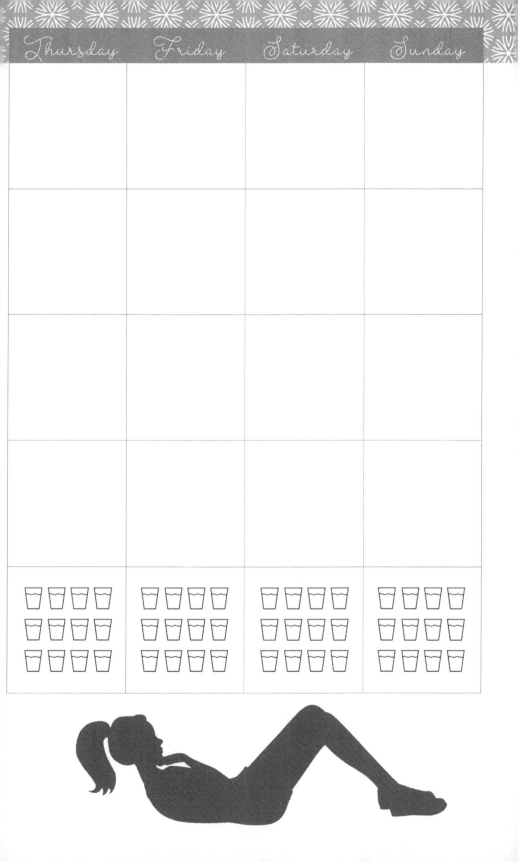

Plan
AHEAD

Date: _____ _____ _____   TO _____ _____ _____

	Current	Goal
WEIGHT:		
BODY FAT %:		
ENERGY LEVEL:		
OTHER:		

This week's plan

WORK OUT SCHEDULE: **S   M   T   W   T   F   S**

NUTRITION: _____

_____

_____

GOALS: _____

_____

_____

Reward

_____

_____

_____

_____

_____

Notes

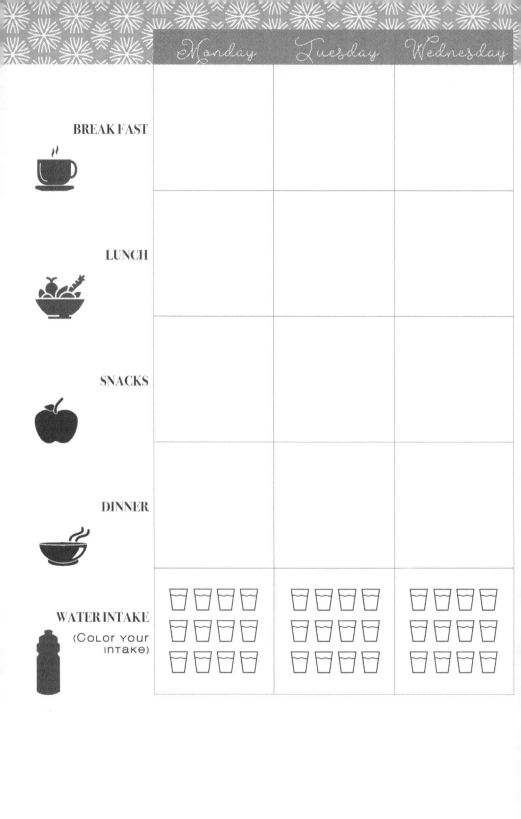

	Monday	Tuesday	Wednesday
BREAKFAST			
LUNCH			
SNACKS			
DINNER			
WATER INTAKE (Color your intake)			

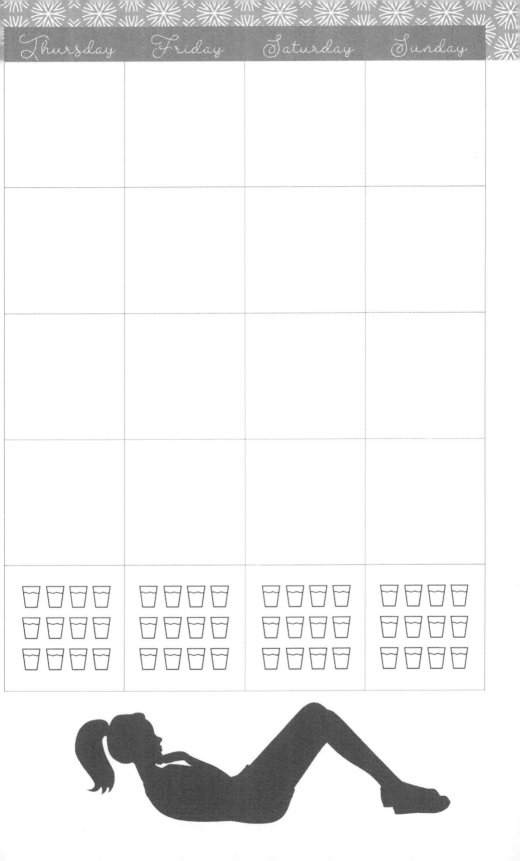

Thursday	Friday	Saturday	Sunday

Strength Training

Exercise	Reps.	Sets	Focus

Notes

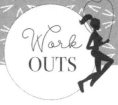

Work
OUTS

CARDIO: Exercise · · · · · · · · · · · · · · · Duration · · · Cals. Burned

_____ _____ _____

_____ _____ _____

_____ _____ _____

STRETCH: Cool-down · TIME

_____ _____

_____ _____

_____ _____

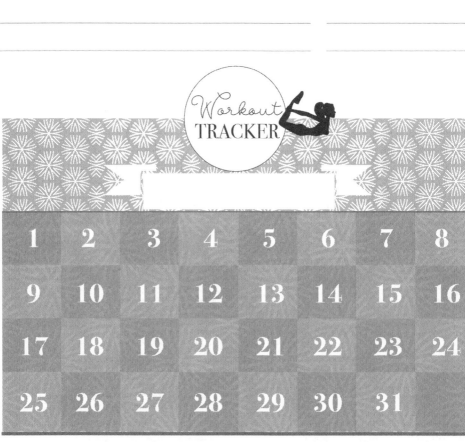

Workout
TRACKER

1	2	3	4	5	6	7	8
9	10	11	12	13	14	15	16
17	18	19	20	21	22	23	24
25	26	27	28	29	30	31	

Habits TRACKER

Everyday habits

1		4	
2		5	
3		6	

	1	2	3	4	5	6		1	2	3	4	5	6
1							17						
2							18						
3							19						
4							20						
5							21						
6							22						
7							23						
8							24						
9							25						
10							26						
11							27						
12							28						
13							29						
14							30						
15							31						
16													

Plan
AHEAD

Date: _____ _____ _____   TO _____ _____ _____

	Current	Goal
Weight:		
Body fat %:		
Energy Level:		
Other:		

This week's plan

Work out schedule: **S   M   T   W   T   F   S**

Nutrition: _____
_____
_____

Goals: _____
_____
_____

Reward

_____
_____
_____
_____
_____

Notes

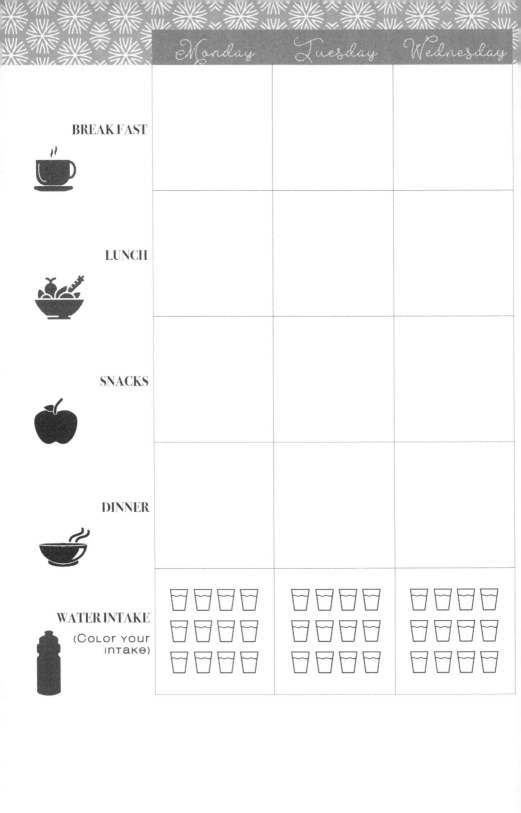

	Monday	Tuesday	Wednesday
BREAKFAST			
LUNCH			
SNACKS			
DINNER			
WATER INTAKE (Color your intake)			

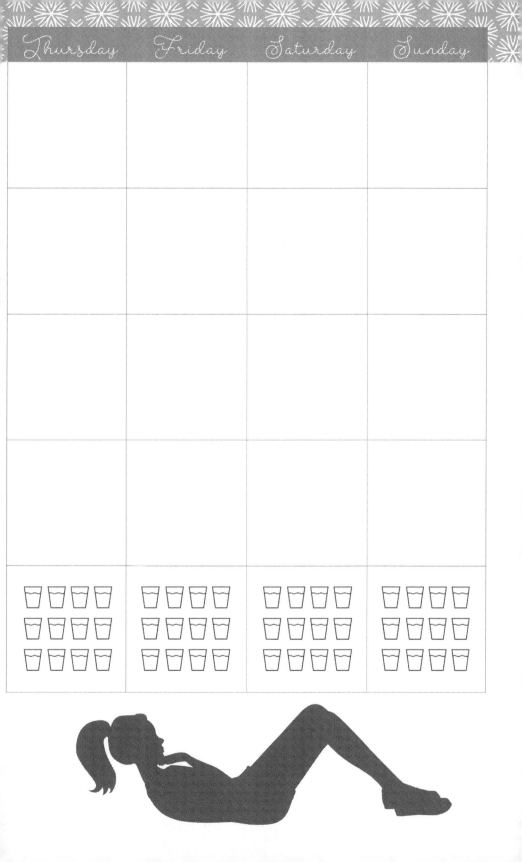

Plan
AHEAD

Date: _____ _____ _____ to _____ _____ _____

	Current	Goal
Weight:		
Body fat %:		
Energy Level:		
Other:		

This week's plan

Work out schedule: S M T W T F S

Nutrition: _____

_____

Goals: _____

_____

_____

Reward

_____

_____

_____

_____

Notes

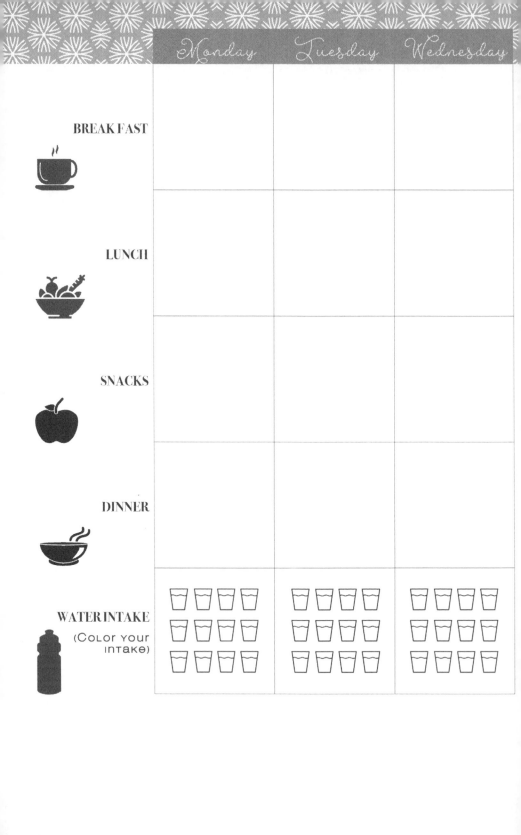

	Monday	Tuesday	Wednesday
BREAKFAST			
LUNCH			
SNACKS			
DINNER			
WATER INTAKE (Color your intake)			

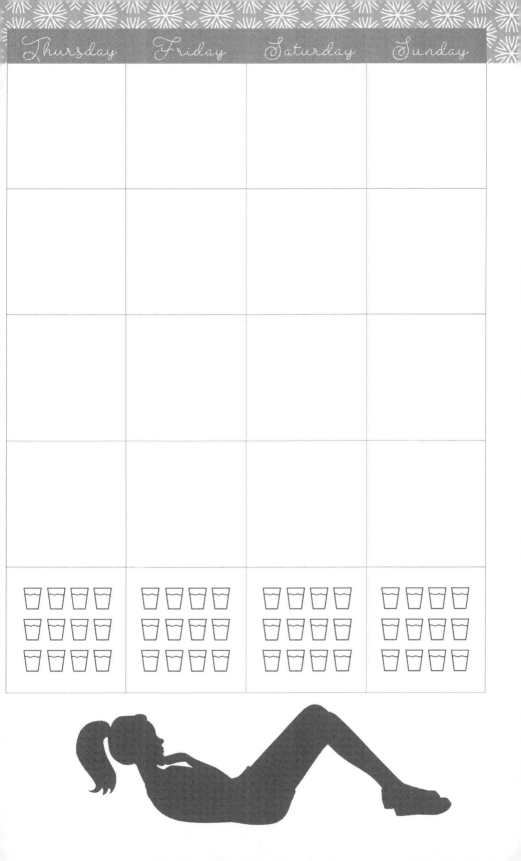

Thursday	Friday	Saturday	Sunday

Plan AHEAD

Date: _____ _____ _____ TO _____ _____ _____

	Current	Goal
Weight:		
Body fat %:		
Energy Level:		
Other:		

This week's plan

Work out schedule: **S M T W T F S**

Nutrition: _____

_____

_____

Goals: _____

_____

_____

Reward

_____

_____

_____

_____

_____

Notes

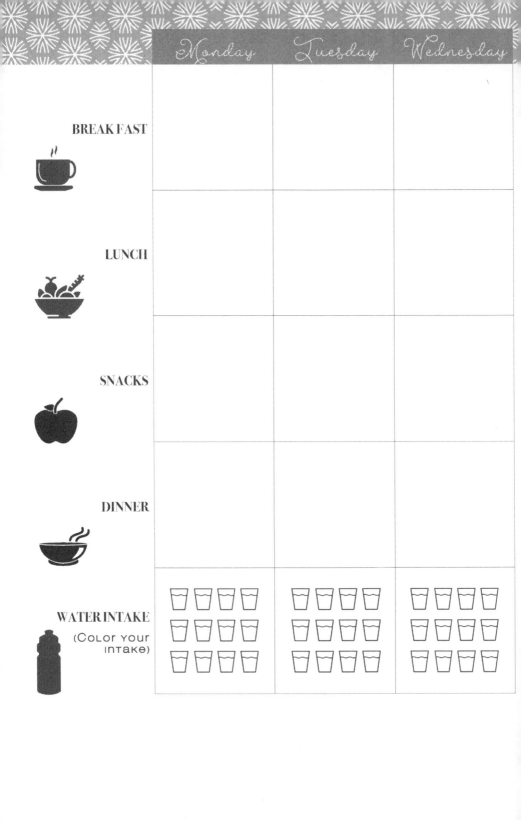

	Monday	Tuesday	Wednesday
BREAK FAST			
LUNCH			
SNACKS			
DINNER			
WATER INTAKE (Color your intake)			

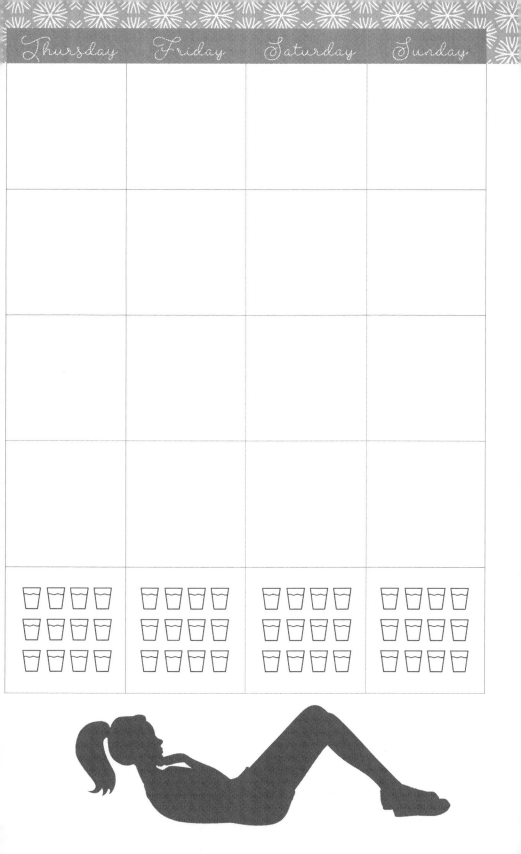

Thursday	Friday	Saturday	Sunday

Date: _____ _____ _____   TO _____ _____ _____

	Current	Goal
Weight:		
Body fat %:		
Energy Level:		
Other:		

This week's plan

Work out schedule: **S   M   T   W   T   F   S**

Nutrition:

_____

_____

_____

Goals:

_____

_____

_____

Reward

_____

_____

_____

_____

_____

Notes

_____
_____
_____
_____
_____
_____
_____
_____
_____
_____
_____
_____
_____
_____
_____
_____
_____
_____
_____
_____
_____
_____

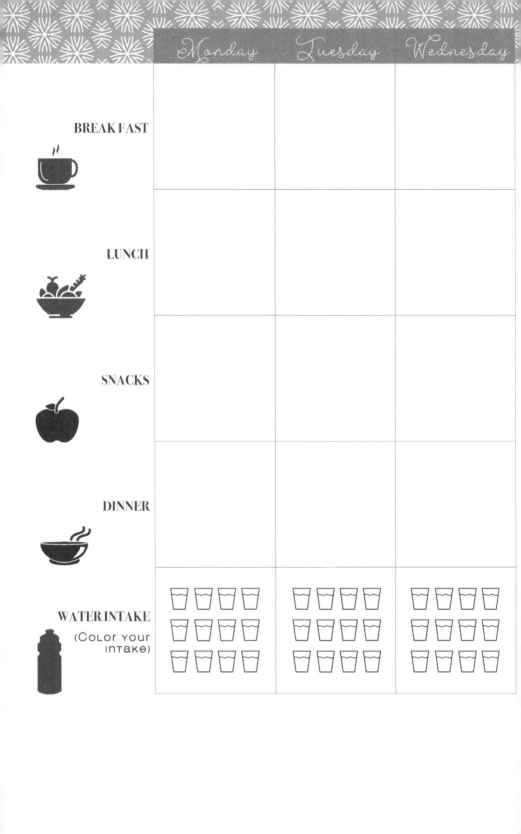

Thursday	Friday	Saturday	Sunday
🥛🥛🥛🥛 🥛🥛🥛🥛 🥛🥛🥛🥛	🥛🥛🥛🥛 🥛🥛🥛🥛 🥛🥛🥛🥛	🥛🥛🥛🥛 🥛🥛🥛🥛 🥛🥛🥛🥛	🥛🥛🥛🥛 🥛🥛🥛🥛 🥛🥛🥛🥛

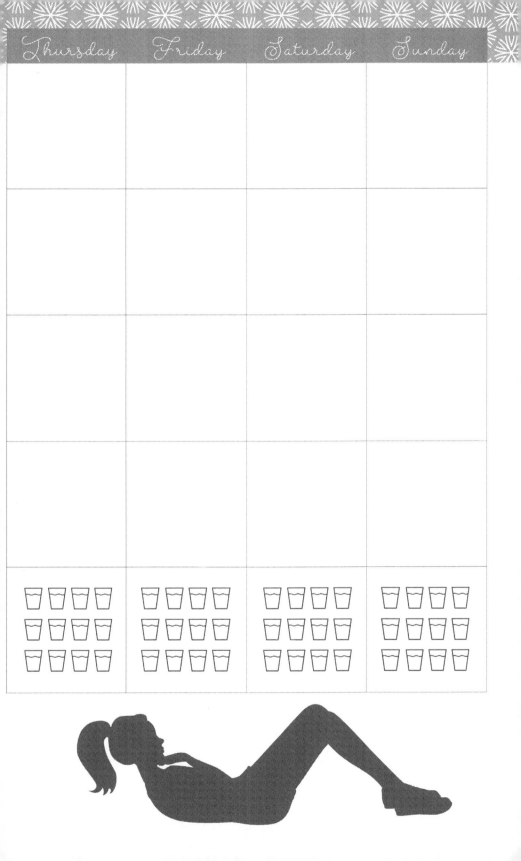

Strength Training

Exercise	Reps.	Sets	Focus

Notes

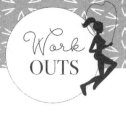

Work OUTS

CARDIO: Exercise   Duration   Cals. Burned

_____   _____   _____

_____   _____   _____

_____   _____   _____

STRETCH: Cool-down   TIME

_____   _____

_____   _____

_____   _____

Workout TRACKER

1	2	3	4	5	6	7	8
9	10	11	12	13	14	15	16
17	18	19	20	21	22	23	24
25	26	27	28	29	30	31	

Habits TRACKER

Everyday habits

1		4	
2		5	
3		6	

	1	2	3	4	5	6		1	2	3	4	5	6
1							17						
2							18						
3							19						
4							20						
5							21						
6							22						
7							23						
8							24						
9							25						
10							26						
11							27						
12							28						
13							29						
14							30						
15							31						
16													

Plan
AHEAD

Date: _____ _____ _____ to _____ _____ _____

	Current	Goal
Weight:		
Body fat %:		
Energy Level:		
Other:		

This week's plan

Work out schedule: S M T W T F S

Nutrition: _____
_____
_____

Goals: _____
_____
_____

Reward

_____
_____
_____
_____
_____

Notes

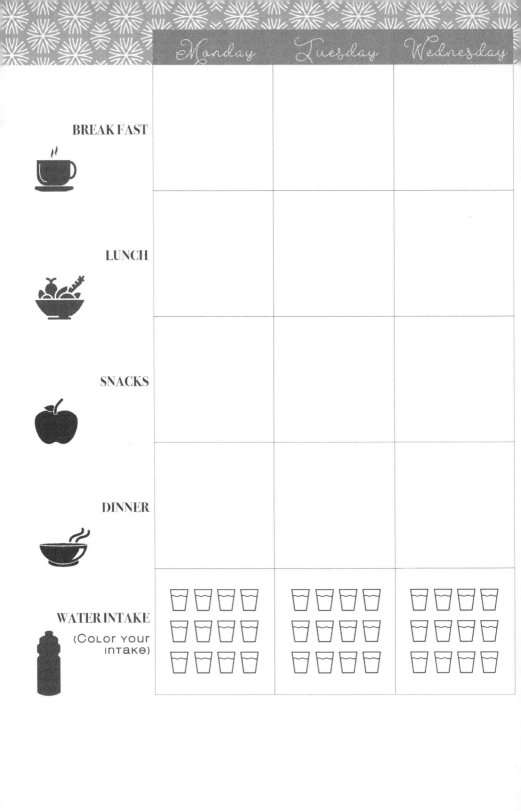

	Monday	Tuesday	Wednesday
BREAK FAST			
LUNCH			
SNACKS			
DINNER			
WATER INTAKE (Color your intake)			

Thursday	Friday	Saturday	Sunday

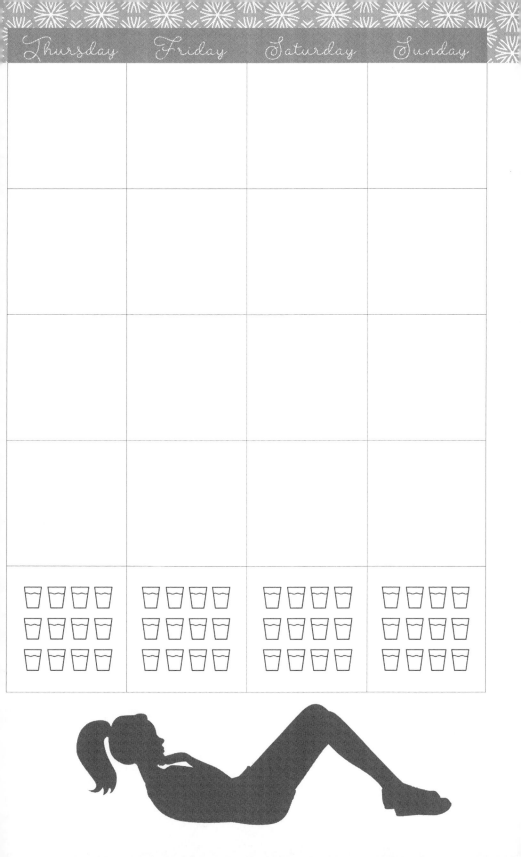

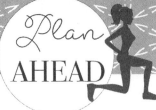

Plan
AHEAD

Date: _____ TO _____

	Current	Goal
Weight:		
Body fat %:		
Energy Level:		
Other:		

This week's plan

Work out schedule: **S   M   T   W   T   F   S**

Nutrition: _____

_____

_____

Goals: _____

_____

_____

Reward

_____

_____

_____

_____

_____

Notes

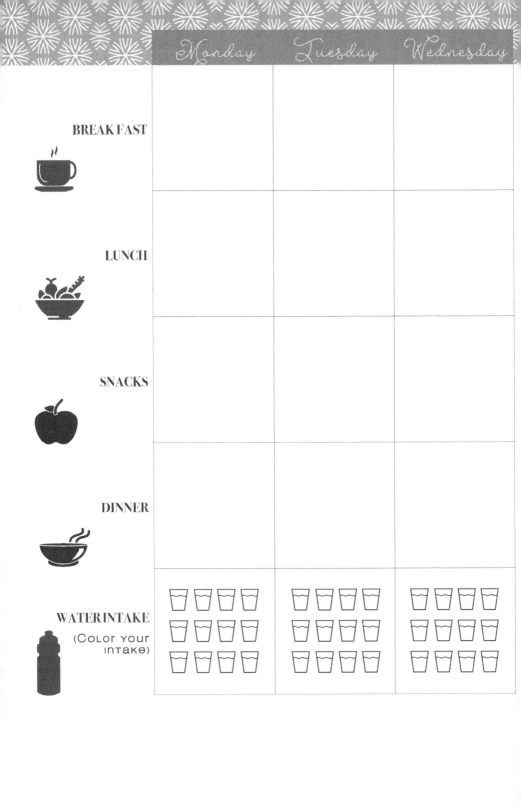

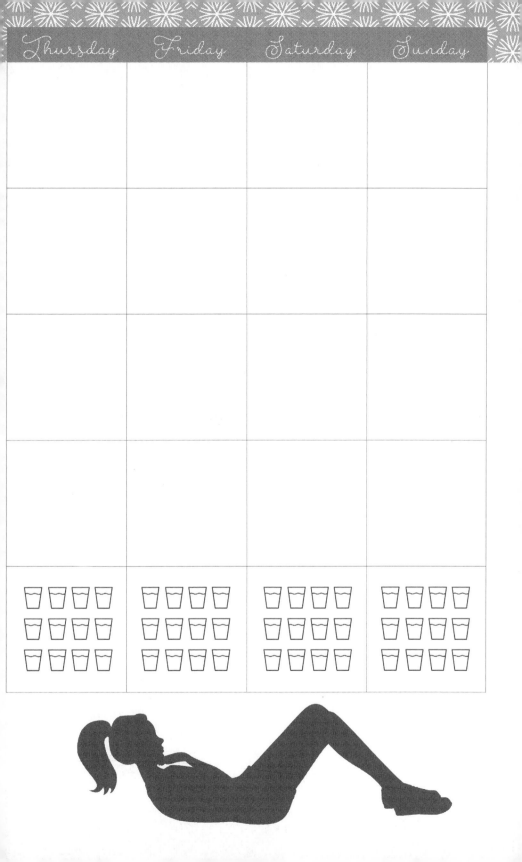

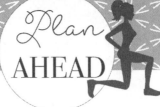

Plan AHEAD

Date: _____ _____ _____   TO _____ _____ _____

	Current	Goal
Weight:		
Body fat %:		
Energy Level:		
Other:		

This week's plan

Work out schedule: **S   M   T   W   T   F   S**

Nutrition: _____
_____
_____

Goals: _____
_____
_____

Reward

_____
_____
_____
_____
_____

Notes

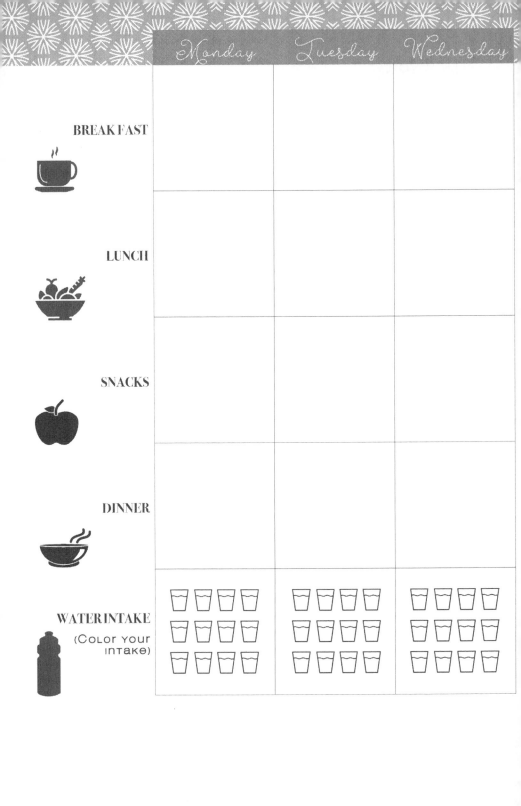

	Monday	Tuesday	Wednesday
BREAKFAST			
LUNCH			
SNACKS			
DINNER			
WATER INTAKE (Color your intake)			

Thursday	Friday	Saturday	Sunday

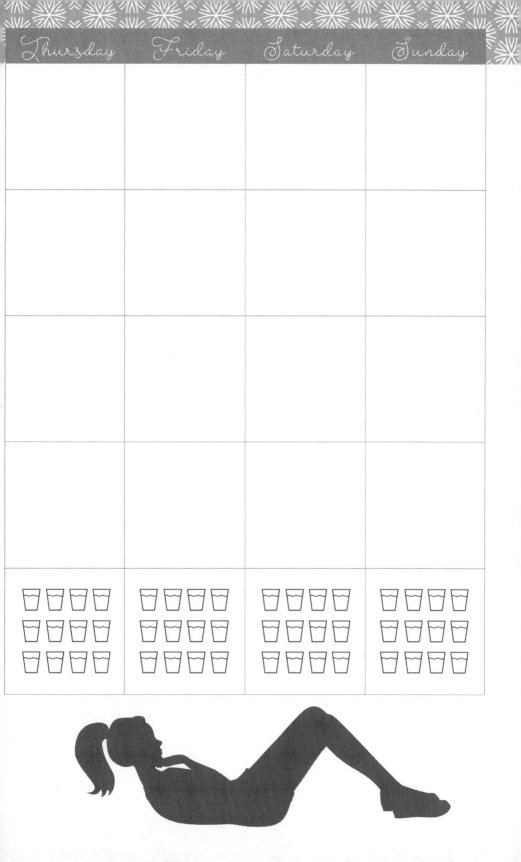

Plan AHEAD

Date: _____ TO _____

	Current	Goal
Weight:		
Body fat %:		
Energy Level:		
Other:		

This week's plan

Work out schedule: S M T W T F S

Nutrition: _____
_____
_____

Goals: _____
_____
_____
_____

Reward

_____
_____
_____
_____
_____

Notes

_____

_____

_____

_____

_____

_____

_____

_____

_____

_____

_____

_____

_____

_____

_____

_____

_____

_____

_____

_____

_____

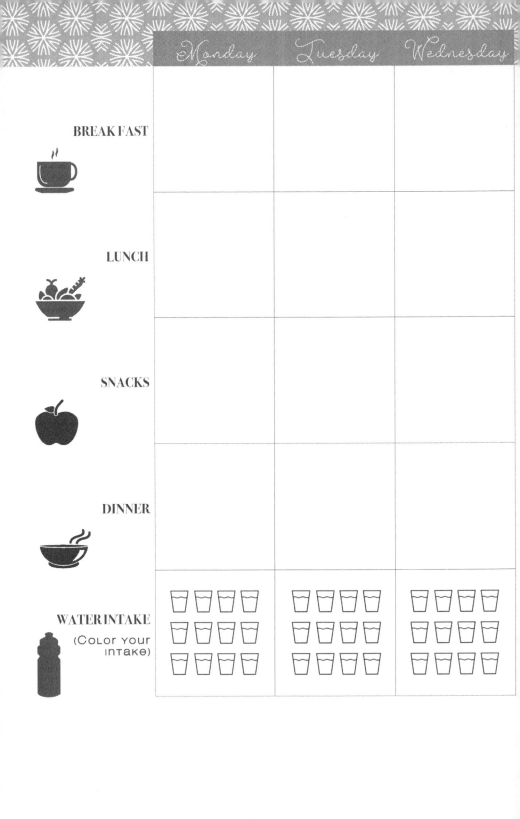

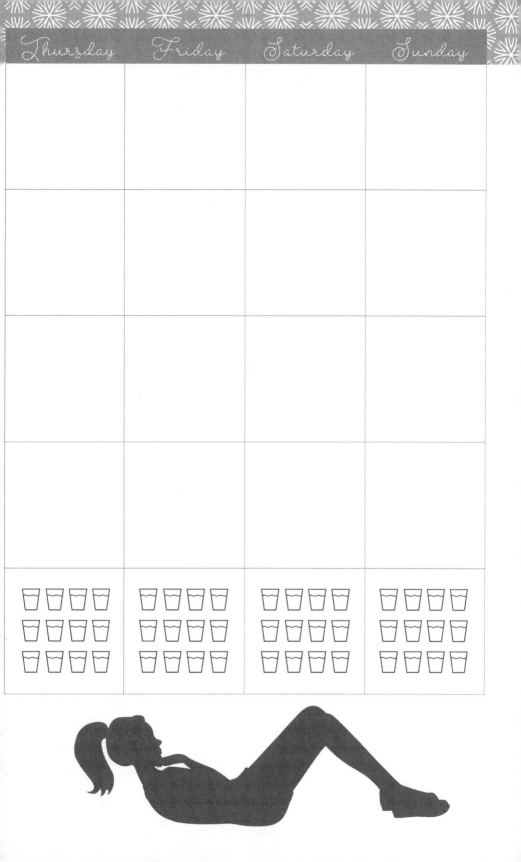

Thursday	Friday	Saturday	Sunday

Work
OUTS

Strength Training

Exercise	Reps.	Sets	Focus

Notes

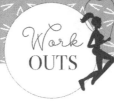

Work
OUTS

CARDIO: Exercise   Duration   Cals. Burned

_____   _____   _____

_____   _____   _____

_____   _____   _____

STRETCH: Cool-down   TIME

_____   _____

_____   _____

_____   _____

Workout
TRACKER

1	2	3	4	5	6	7	8
9	10	11	12	13	14	15	16
17	18	19	20	21	22	23	24
25	26	27	28	29	30	31	

Habits TRACKER

Everyday habits

1 _____ 4 _____

2 _____ 5 _____

3 _____ 6 _____

	1	2	3	4	5	6		1	2	3	4	5	6
1							17						
2							18						
3							19						
4							20						
5							21						
6							22						
7							23						
8							24						
9							25						
10							26						
11							27						
12							28						
13							29						
14							30						
15							31						
16													

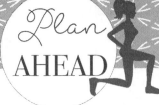

Plan AHEAD

Date: _____ _____ _____ to _____ _____ _____

	Current	Goal
Weight:	_____	_____
Body fat %:	_____	_____
Energy Level:	_____	_____
Other:	_____	_____

This week's plan

Work out schedule: **S   M   T   W   T   F   S**

Nutrition: _____

_____

_____

Goals: _____

_____

_____

Reward

_____

_____

_____

_____

Notes

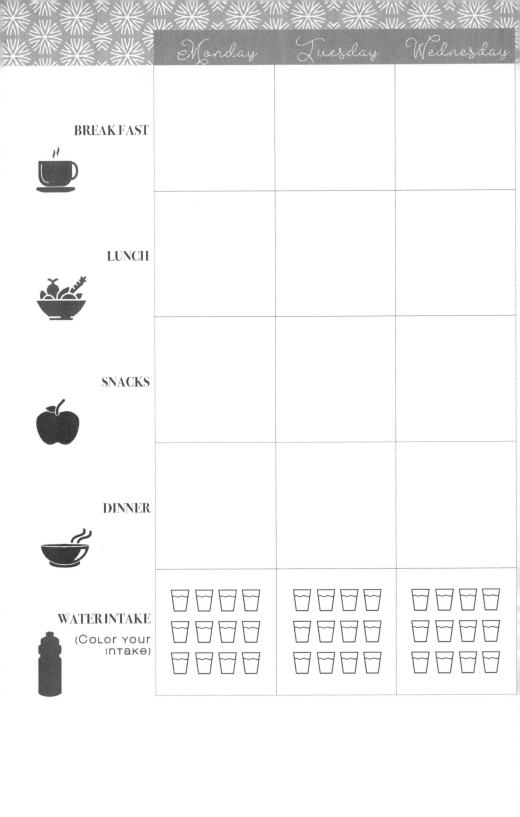

	Monday	Tuesday	Wednesday
BREAKFAST			
LUNCH			
SNACKS			
DINNER			
WATER INTAKE (Color your intake)			

Thursday	Friday	Saturday	Sunday

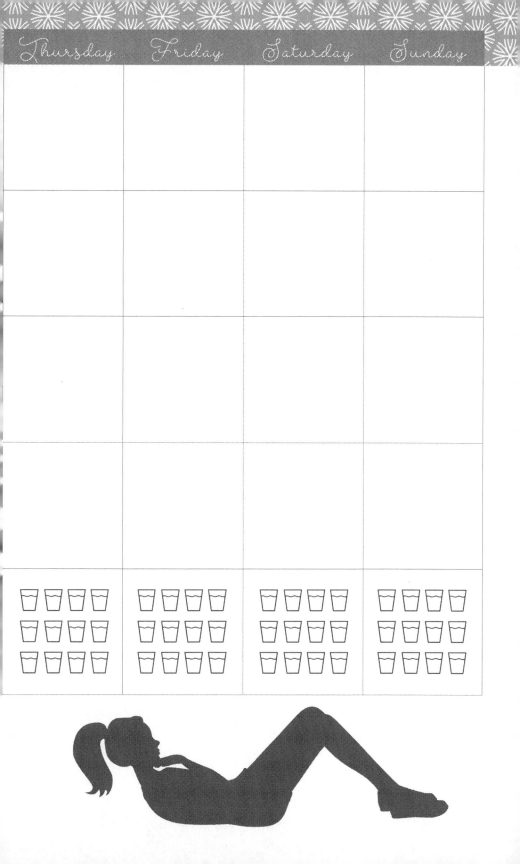

Plan AHEAD

Date: _____ _____ _____ to _____ _____ _____

	Current	Goal
Weight:		
Body fat %:		
Energy Level:		
Other:		

This week's plan

Work out schedule: S M T W T F S

Nutrition: _____

_____

_____

Goals: _____

_____

_____

Reward

_____

_____

_____

_____

_____

Notes

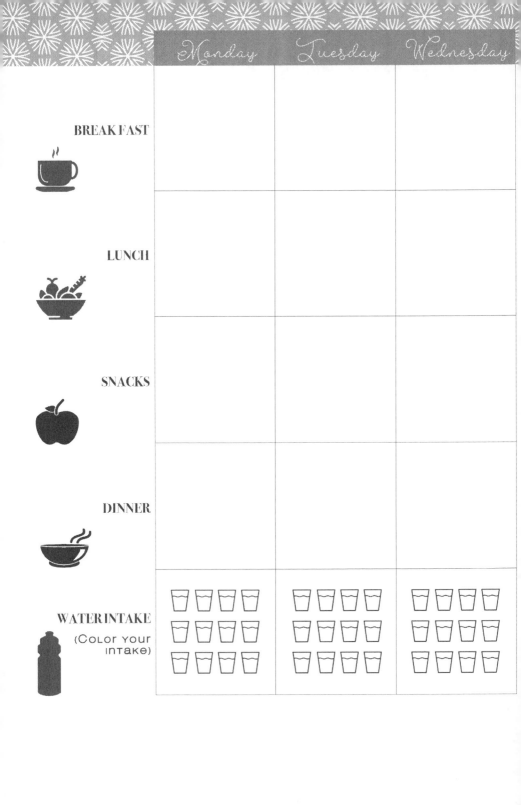

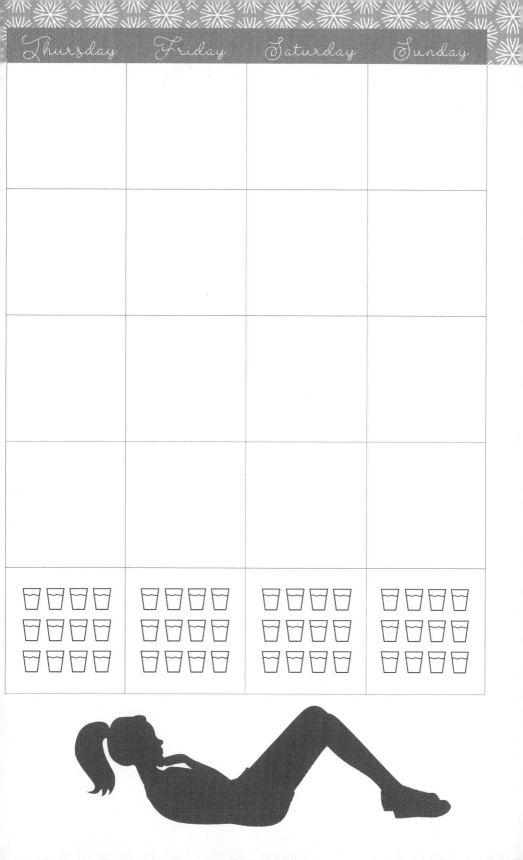

Thursday	Friday	Saturday	Sunday

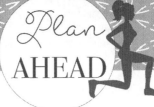

Plan
AHEAD

Date: _____ TO _____

	Current	Goal
Weight:		
Body fat %:		
Energy Level:		
Other:		

This week's plan

Work out schedule: S   M   T   W   T   F   S

Nutrition: _____

_____

_____

Goals: _____

_____

_____

Reward

_____

_____

_____

_____

_____

Notes

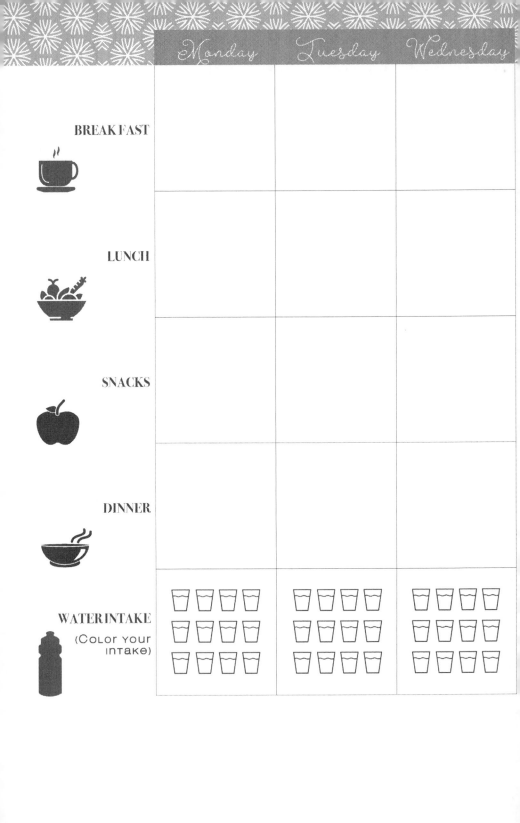

	Monday	Tuesday	Wednesday
BREAKFAST			
LUNCH			
SNACKS			
DINNER			
WATER INTAKE (Color your intake)			

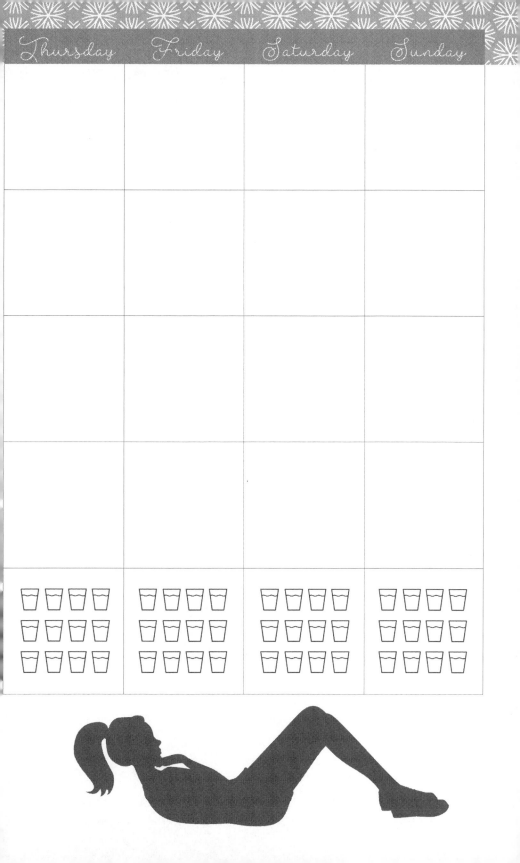

Thursday	Friday	Saturday	Sunday

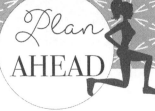

Plan AHEAD

Date: _____ _____ _____ TO _____ _____ _____

	Current	Goal
Weight:		
Body fat %:		
Energy Level:		
Other:		

This week's plan

Work out schedule: S M T W T F S

Nutrition: _____
_____
_____

Goals: _____
_____
_____

Reward

_____
_____
_____
_____

Notes

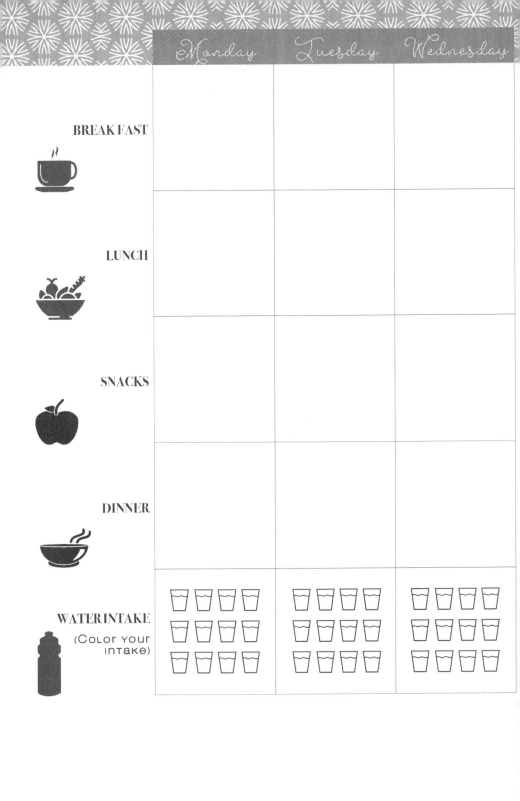

Thursday	Friday	Saturday	Sunday

Strength Training

Exercise	Reps.	Sets	Focus

Notes

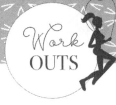

Work
OUTS

CARDIO: Exercise   Duration   Cals. Burned

_____   _____   _____

_____   _____   _____

_____   _____   _____

STRETCH: Cool-down   TIME

_____   _____

_____   _____

_____   _____

Workout
TRACKER

1	2	3	4	5	6	7	8
9	10	11	12	13	14	15	16
17	18	19	20	21	22	23	24
25	26	27	28	29	30	31	

Everyday habits

1		4	
2		5	
3		6	

	1	2	3	4	5	6		1	2	3	4	5	6
1							17						
2							18						
3							19						
4							20						
5							21						
6							22						
7							23						
8							24						
9							25						
10							26						
11							27						
12							28						
13							29						
14							30						
15							31						
16													

Plan
AHEAD

Date: _____ TO _____

	Current	Goal
Weight:		
Body fat %:		
Energy Level:		
Other:		

This week's plan

Work out schedule: S   M   T   W   T   F   S

Nutrition: _____

_____

Goals: _____

_____

_____

Reward

_____

_____

_____

_____

_____

Notes

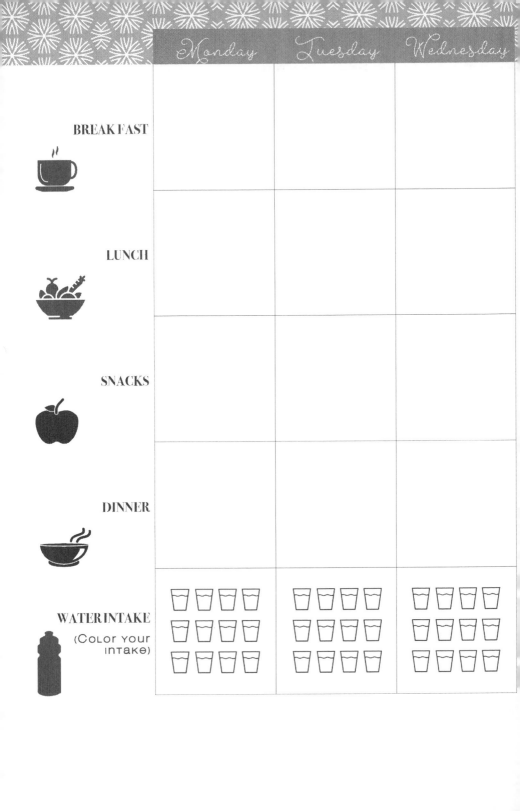

	Monday	Tuesday	Wednesday
BREAKFAST			
LUNCH			
SNACKS			
DINNER			
WATER INTAKE (Color your intake)			

Thursday	Friday	Saturday	Sunday

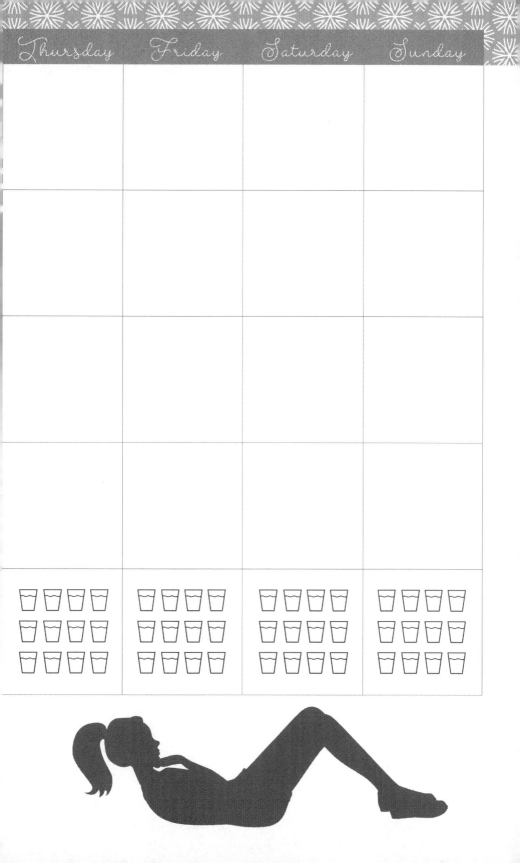

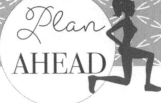

Plan AHEAD

Date: _____ _____ _____   TO _____ _____ _____

	Current	Goal
Weight:		
Body fat %:		
Energy Level:		
Other:		

This week's plan

Work out schedule: **S   M   T   W   T   F   S**

Nutrition: _____
_____
_____

Goals: _____
_____
_____

Reward

_____
_____
_____
_____
_____

Notes

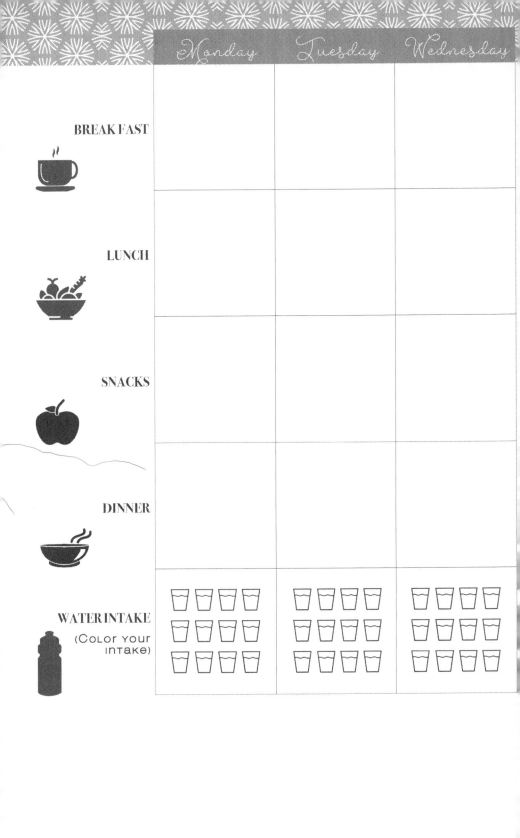

	Monday	Tuesday	Wednesday
BREAKFAST			
LUNCH			
SNACKS			
DINNER			
WATER INTAKE (Color your intake)			

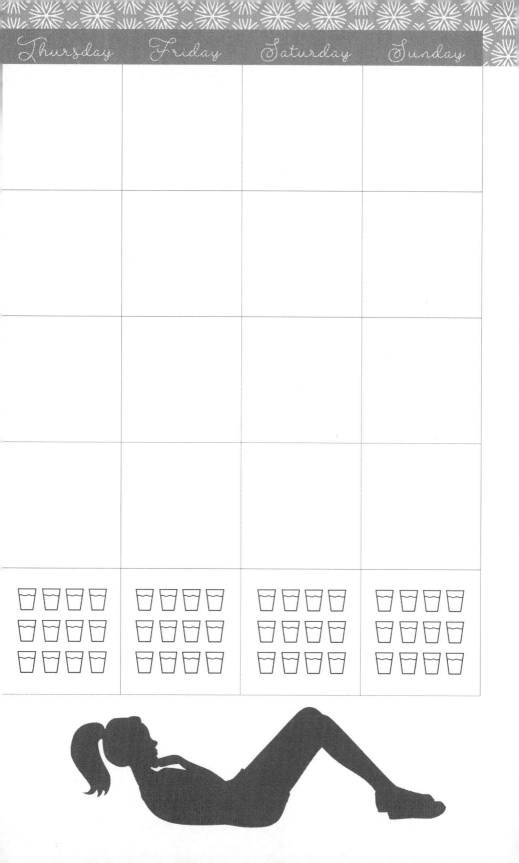

Thursday	Friday	Saturday	Sunday

Plan
AHEAD

Date: _____ _____ _____ TO _____ _____ _____

	Current	Goal
Weight:		
Body fat %:		
Energy Level:		
Other:		

This week's plan

Work out schedule: **S   M   T   W   T   F   S**

Nutrition: _____

_____

_____

Goals: _____

_____

_____

Reward

_____

_____

_____

_____

_____

Notes

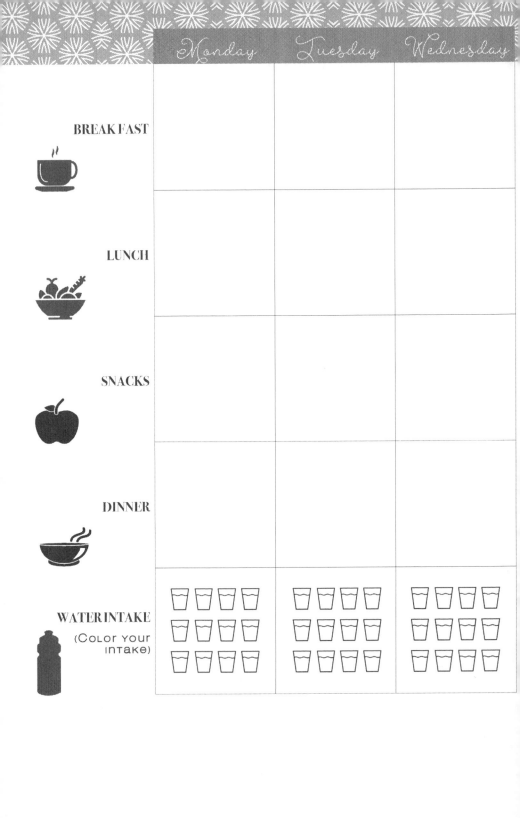

	Monday	Tuesday	Wednesday
BREAKFAST			
LUNCH			
SNACKS			
DINNER			
WATER INTAKE (Color your intake)			

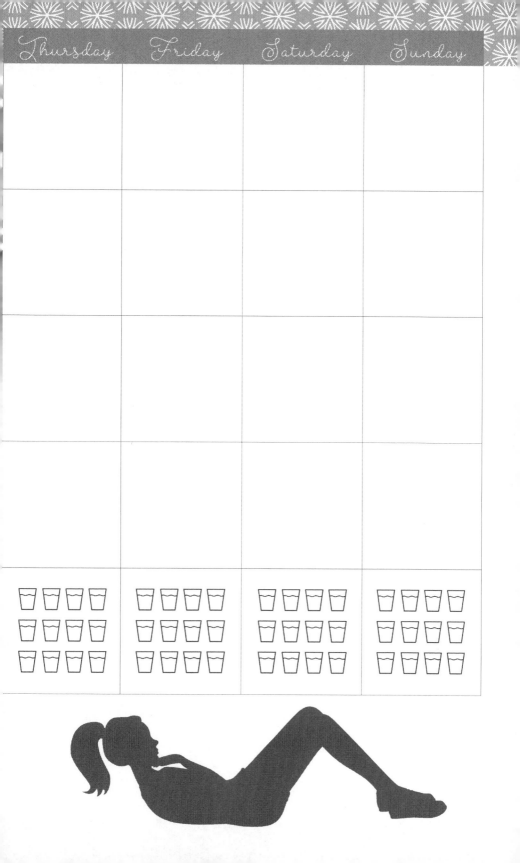

Thursday	Friday	Saturday	Sunday

Plan
AHEAD

Date: _____ _____ _____   TO _____ _____ _____

	Current	Goal
Weight:	_____	_____
Body fat %:	_____	_____
Energy Level:	_____	_____
Other:	_____	_____

This week's plan

Work out schedule: **S   M   T   W   T   F   S**

Nutrition:

_____

_____

_____

Goals:

_____

_____

_____

Reward

_____

_____

_____

_____

_____

Notes

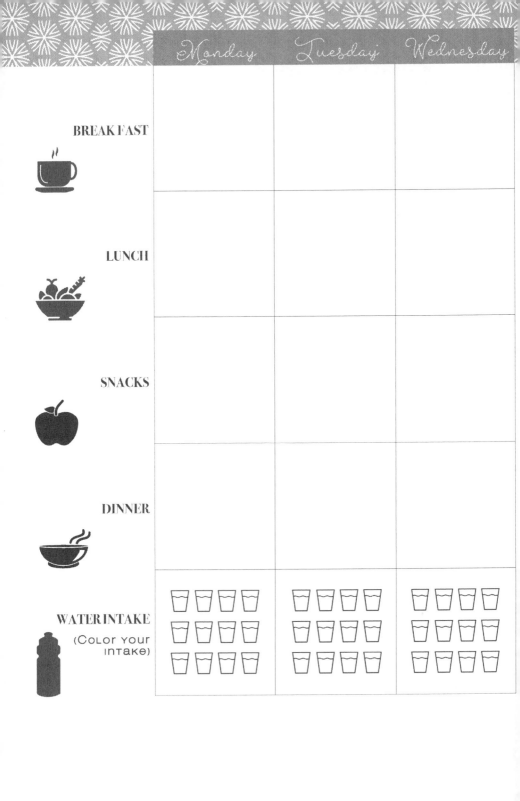

	Monday	Tuesday	Wednesday
BREAKFAST			
LUNCH			
SNACKS			
DINNER			
WATER INTAKE (Color your intake)			

Thursday	Friday	Saturday	Sunday

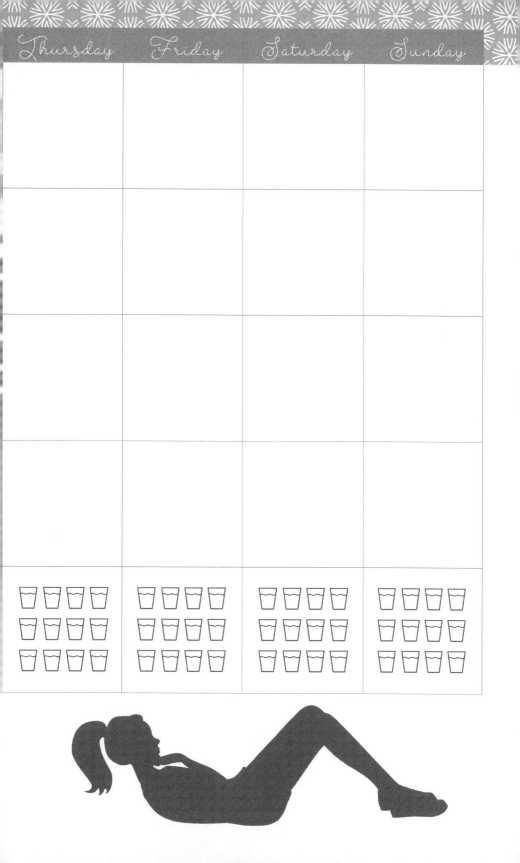

Strength Training

Exercise	Reps.	Sets	Focus

Notes

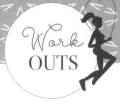

Work OUTS

CARDIO: Exercise   Duration   Cals. Burned

_____   _____   _____

_____   _____   _____

_____   _____   _____

STRETCH: Cool-down   TIME

_____   _____

_____   _____

_____   _____

Workout TRACKER

1	2	3	4	5	6	7	8
9	10	11	12	13	14	15	16
17	18	19	20	21	22	23	24
25	26	27	28	29	30	31	

Habits TRACKER

Everyday habits

1 _____	4 _____
2 _____	5 _____
3 _____	6 _____

	1	2	3	4	5	6		1	2	3	4	5	6
1							17						
2							18						
3							19						
4							20						
5							21						
6							22						
7							23						
8							24						
9							25						
10							26						
11							27						
12							28						
13							29						
14							30						
15							31						
16													

Plan
AHEAD

Date: _____ _____ TO _____ _____

	Current	Goal
Weight:		
Body fat %:		
Energy Level:		
Other:		

This week's plan

Work out schedule: **S M T W T F S**

Nutrition: _____
_____
_____

Goals: _____
_____
_____

Reward

_____
_____
_____
_____
_____

Notes

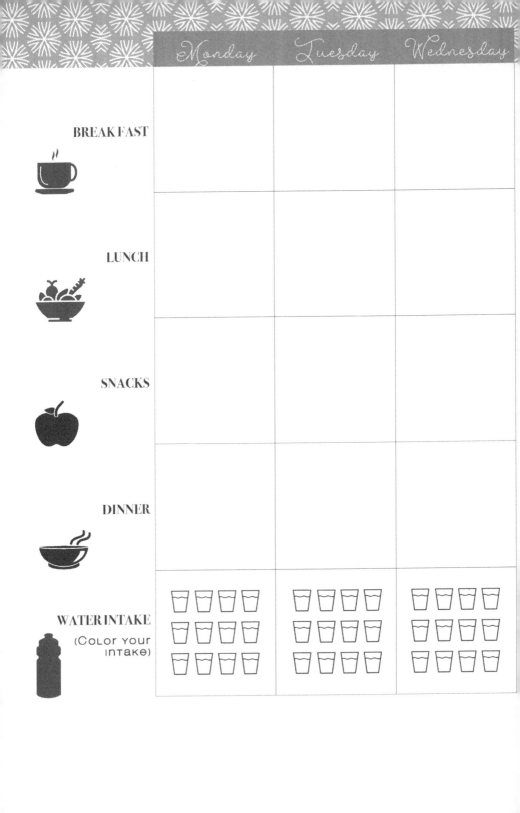

	Monday	Tuesday	Wednesday
BREAKFAST			
LUNCH			
SNACKS			
DINNER			
WATER INTAKE (Color your intake)			

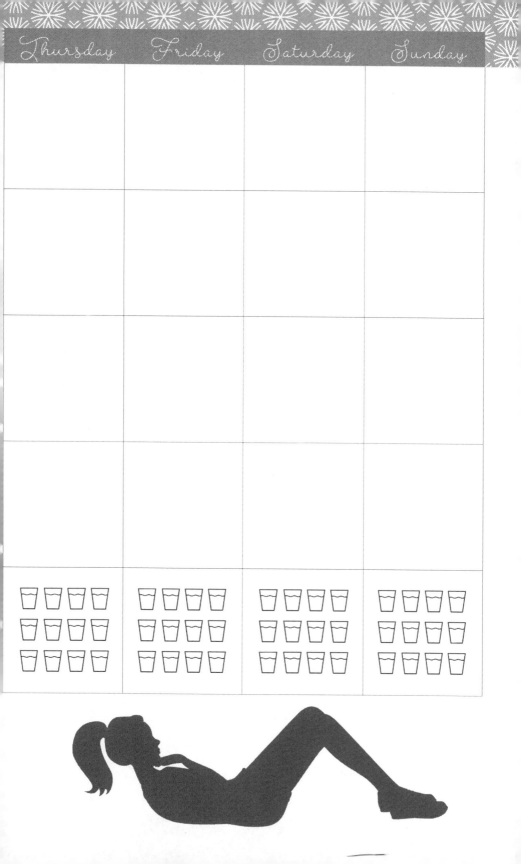

Plan
AHEAD

Date: _____ _____ _____   TO _____ _____ _____

	Current	Goal
Weight:	_____	_____
Body fat %:	_____	_____
Energy Level:	_____	_____
Other:	_____	_____

This week's plan

Work out schedule: **S   M   T   W   T   F   S**

Nutrition: _____
_____
_____

Goals: _____
_____
_____

Reward

_____
_____
_____
_____
_____

Notes

	Monday	Tuesday	Wednesday
BREAKFAST			
LUNCH			
SNACKS			
DINNER			
WATER INTAKE (Color your intake)			

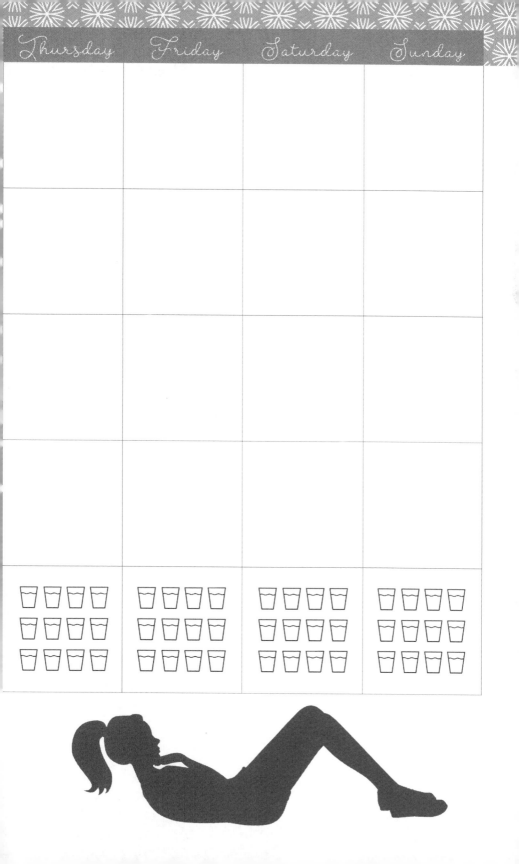

Thursday	Friday	Saturday	Sunday

Plan AHEAD

Date: _____ _____ _____   TO _____ _____ _____

	Current	Goal
Weight:		
Body fat %:		
Energy Level:		
Other:		

This week's plan

Work out schedule: **S   M   T   W   T   F   S**

Nutrition: _____
_____
_____

Goals: _____
_____
_____

Reward

_____
_____
_____
_____
_____

Notes

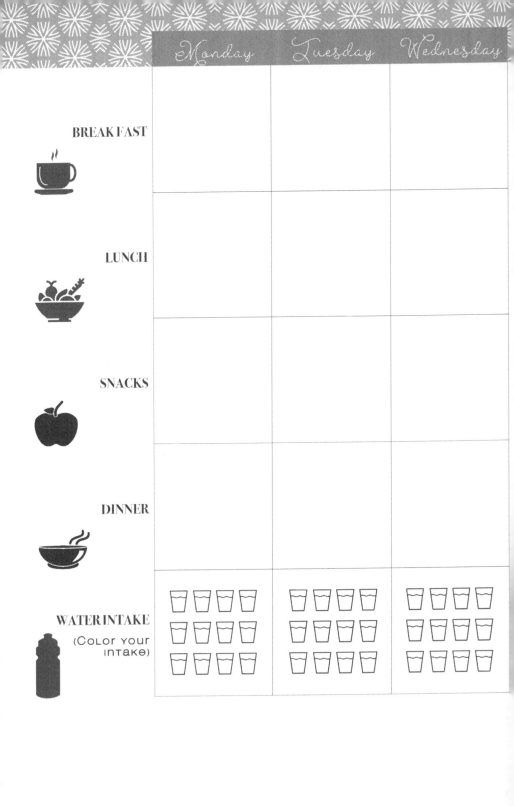

	Monday	Tuesday	Wednesday
BREAKFAST			
LUNCH			
SNACKS			
DINNER			
WATER INTAKE (Color your intake)			

Thursday	Friday	Saturday	Sunday

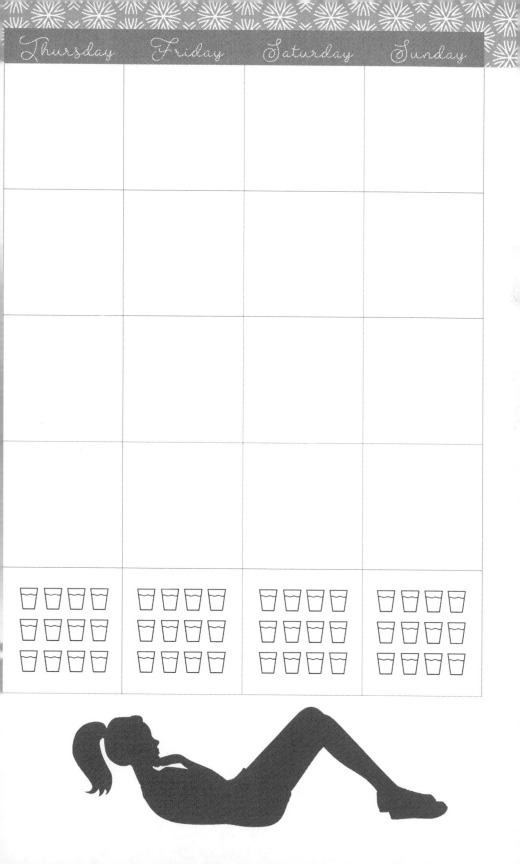

Plan AHEAD

Date: _____ TO _____

	Current	Goal
Weight:		
Body fat %:		
Energy Level:		
Other:		

This week's plan

Work out schedule: **S M T W T F S**

Nutrition: _____

_____

_____

Goals: _____

_____

_____

Reward

_____

_____

_____

_____

_____

Notes

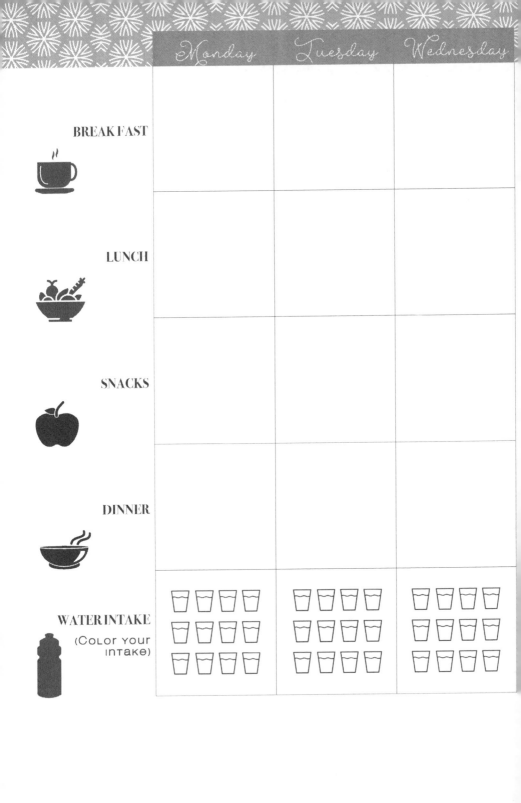

	Monday	Tuesday	Wednesday
BREAK FAST			
LUNCH			
SNACKS			
DINNER			
WATER INTAKE (Color your intake)			

Thursday	Friday	Saturday	Sunday

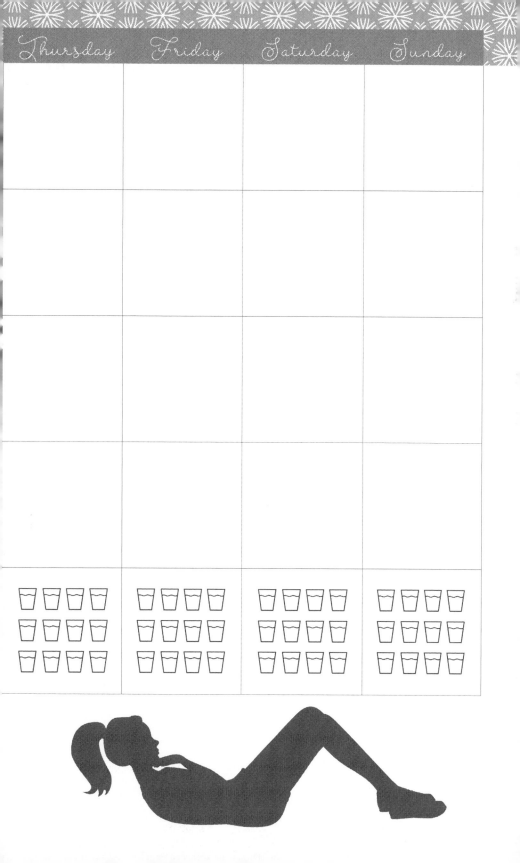

Strength Training

Exercise	Reps.	Sets	Focus

Notes

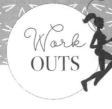

Work
OUTS

CARDIO: Exercise   Duration   Cals. Burned

_____   _____   _____

_____   _____   _____

_____   _____   _____

STRETCH: Cool-down   TIME

_____   _____

_____   _____

_____   _____

Workout
TRACKER

1	2	3	4	5	6	7	8
9	10	11	12	13	14	15	16
17	18	19	20	21	22	23	24
25	26	27	28	29	30	31	

Habits TRACKER

Everyday habits

1		4
2		5
3		6

	1	2	3	4	5	6		1	2	3	4	5	6
1							17						
2							18						
3							19						
4							20						
5							21						
6							22						
7							23						
8							24						
9							25						
10							26						
11							27						
12							28						
13							29						
14							30						
15							31						
16													

Plan
AHEAD

Date: _____ _____ _____   TO _____ _____ _____

	Current	Goal
Weight:		
Body fat %:		
Energy Level:		
Other:		

This week's plan

Work out schedule: S   M   T   W   T   F   S

Nutrition: _____
_____
_____

Goals: _____
_____
_____

Reward

_____
_____
_____
_____
_____

Notes

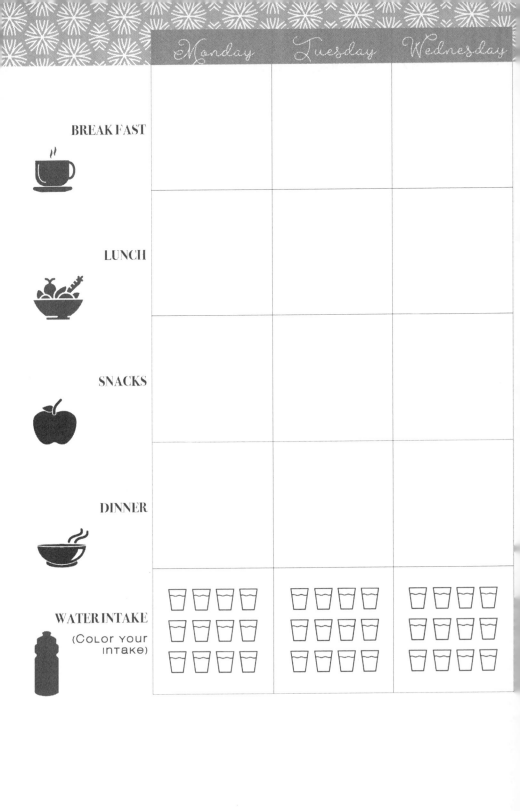

	Monday	Tuesday	Wednesday
BREAKFAST			
LUNCH			
SNACKS			
DINNER			
WATER INTAKE (Color your intake)			

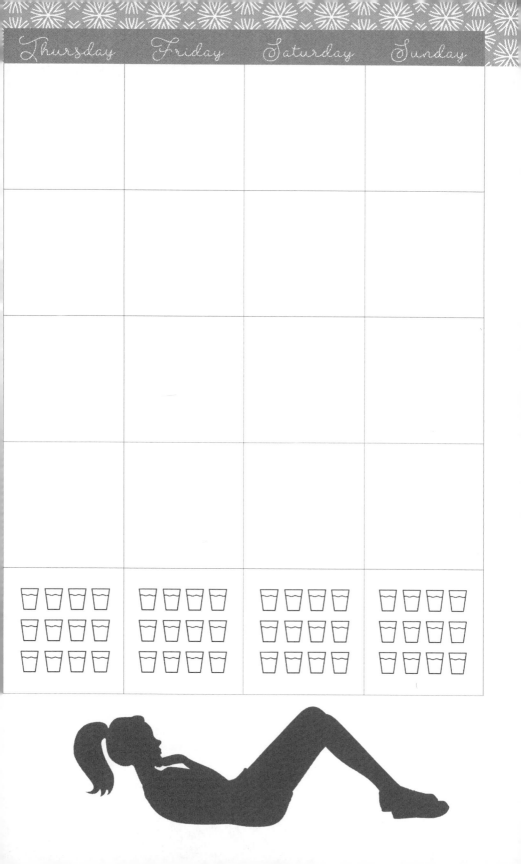

Plan
AHEAD

Date: _____ _____ _____   TO _____ _____ _____

	Current	Goal
Weight:		
Body fat %:		
Energy Level:		
Other:		

This week's plan

Work out schedule: S   M   T   W   T   F   S

Nutrition: _____

_____

_____

Goals: _____

_____

_____

Reward

_____

_____

_____

_____

_____

Notes

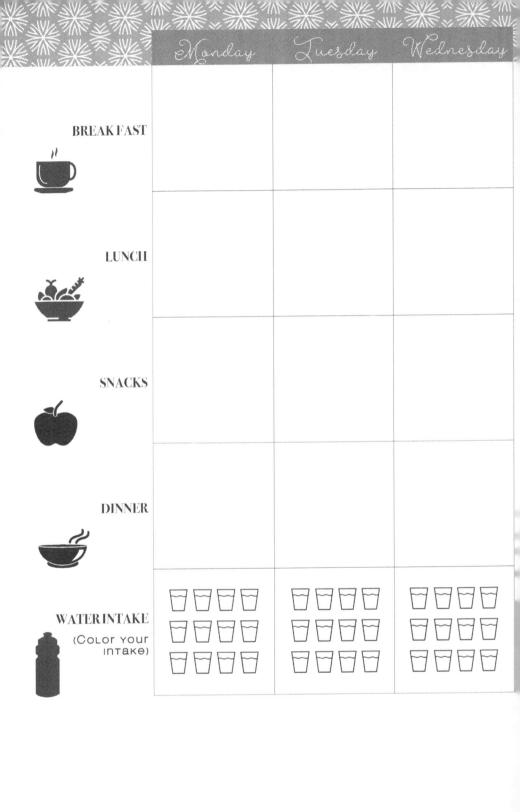

	Monday	Tuesday	Wednesday
BREAKFAST			
LUNCH			
SNACKS			
DINNER			
WATER INTAKE (Color your intake)			

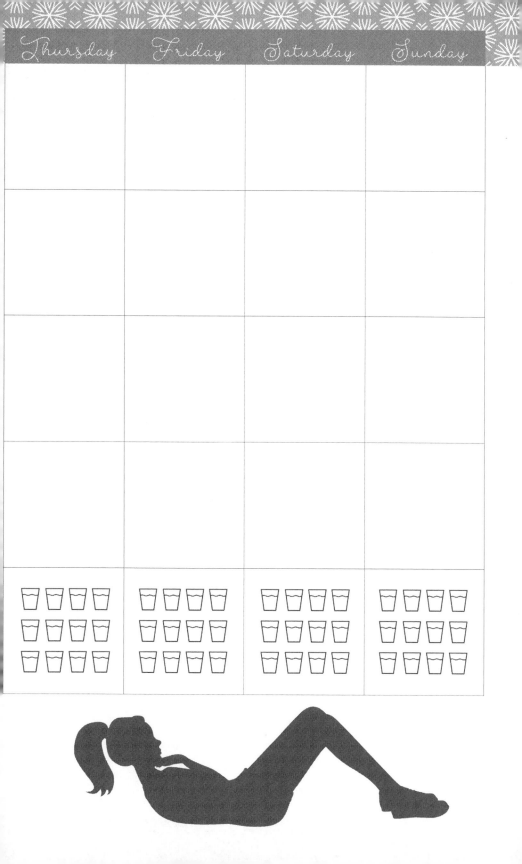

Thursday	Friday	Saturday	Sunday

Plan
AHEAD

Date: _____ _____ _____ TO _____ _____ _____

	Current	Goal
Weight:		
Body fat %:		
Energy Level:		
Other:		

This week's plan

Work out schedule: **S   M   T   W   T   F   S**

Nutrition: _____

_____

_____

Goals: _____

_____

_____

Reward

_____

_____

_____

_____

_____

Notes

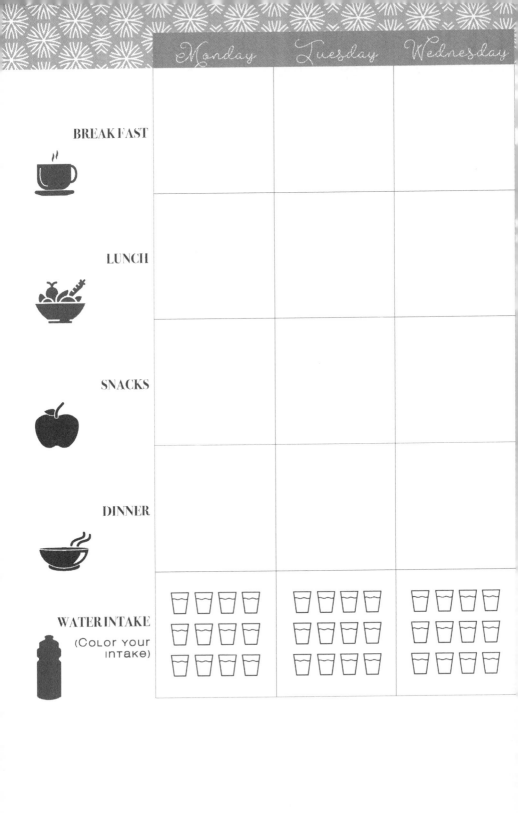

	Monday	Tuesday	Wednesday
BREAKFAST			
LUNCH			
SNACKS			
DINNER			
WATER INTAKE (Color your intake)			

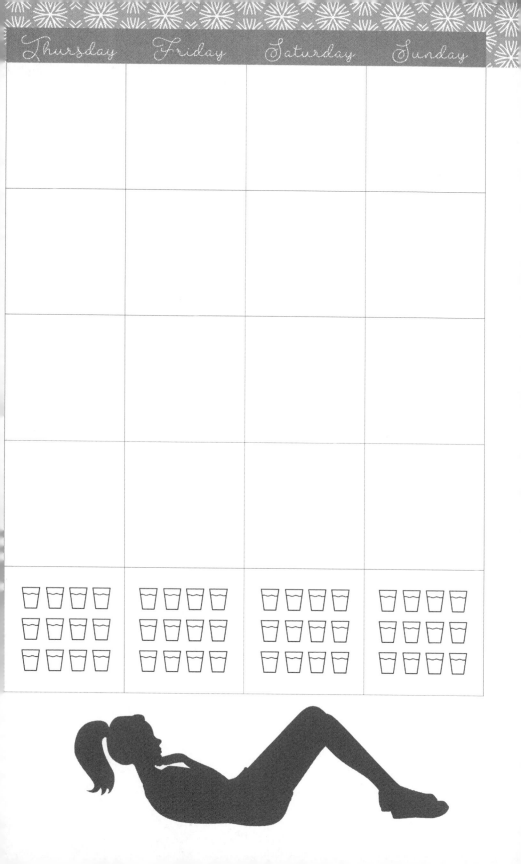

Plan
AHEAD

Date: _____ TO _____

	Current	Goal
Weight:		
Body fat %:		
Energy Level:		
Other:		

This week's plan

Work out schedule: S   M   T   W   T   F   S

Nutrition: _____

_____

Goals: _____

_____

Reward

_____

_____

_____

_____

Notes

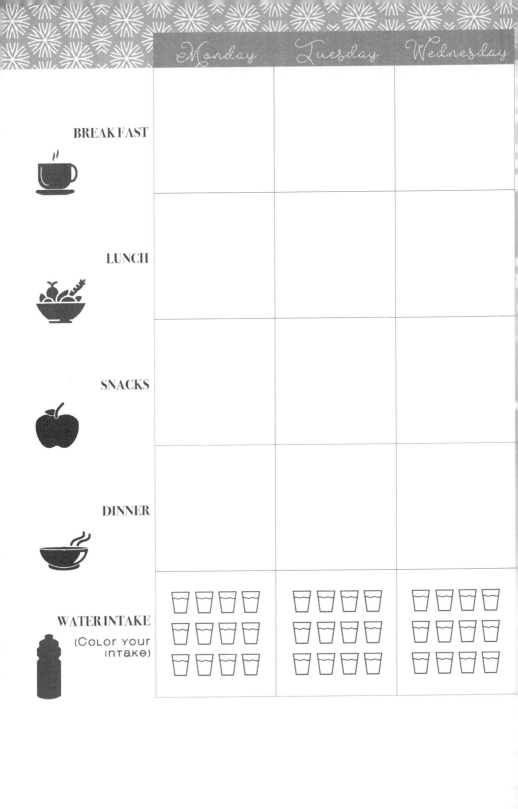

	Monday	Tuesday	Wednesday
BREAKFAST			
LUNCH			
SNACKS			
DINNER			
WATER INTAKE (Color your intake)			

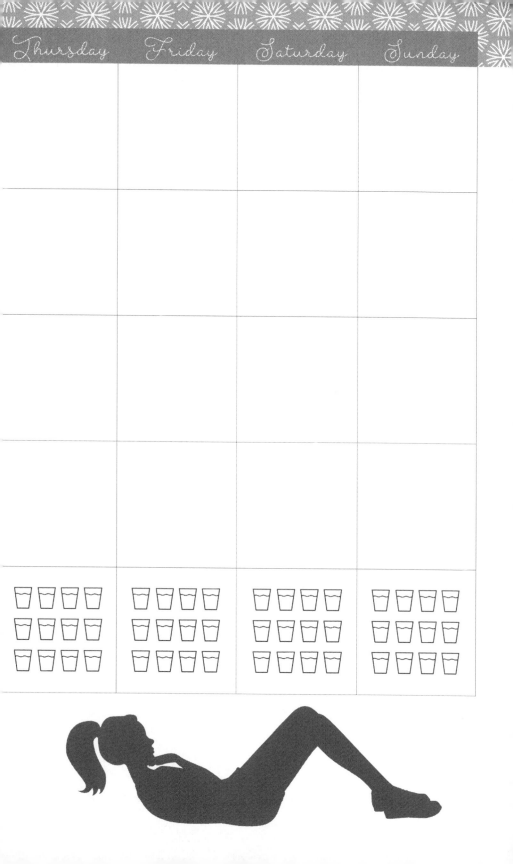

Strength Training

Exercise	Reps.	Sets	Focus

Notes

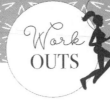

Work
OUTS

CARDIO: Exercise   Duration   Cals. Burned

_____   _____   _____

_____   _____   _____

_____   _____   _____

STRETCH: Cool-down   TIME

_____   _____

_____   _____

_____   _____

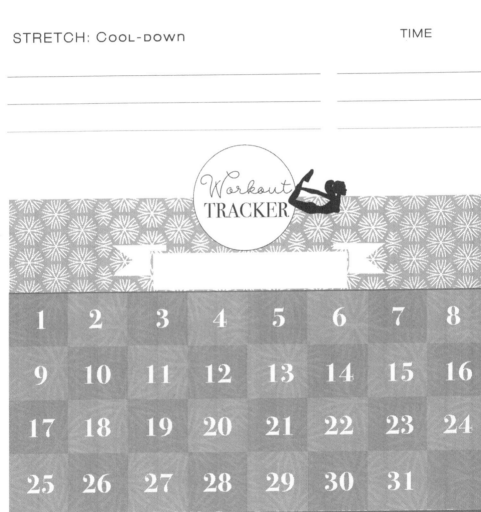

Workout
TRACKER

1	2	3	4	5	6	7	8
9	10	11	12	13	14	15	16
17	18	19	20	21	22	23	24
25	26	27	28	29	30	31	

Habits TRACKER

Everyday habits

1 _____   4 _____
2 _____   5 _____
3 _____   6 _____

	1	2	3	4	5	6		1	2	3	4	5	6
1							17						
2							18						
3							19						
4							20						
5							21						
6							22						
7							23						
8							24						
9							25						
10							26						
11							27						
12							28						
13							29						
14							30						
15							31						
16													

Plan
AHEAD

Date: _____ TO _____

	Current	Goal
Weight:	_____	_____
Body fat %:	_____	_____
Energy Level:	_____	_____
Other:	_____	_____

This week's plan

Work out schedule: **S M T W T F S**

Nutrition: _____

_____

_____

Goals: _____

_____

_____

Reward

_____

_____

_____

_____

_____

Notes

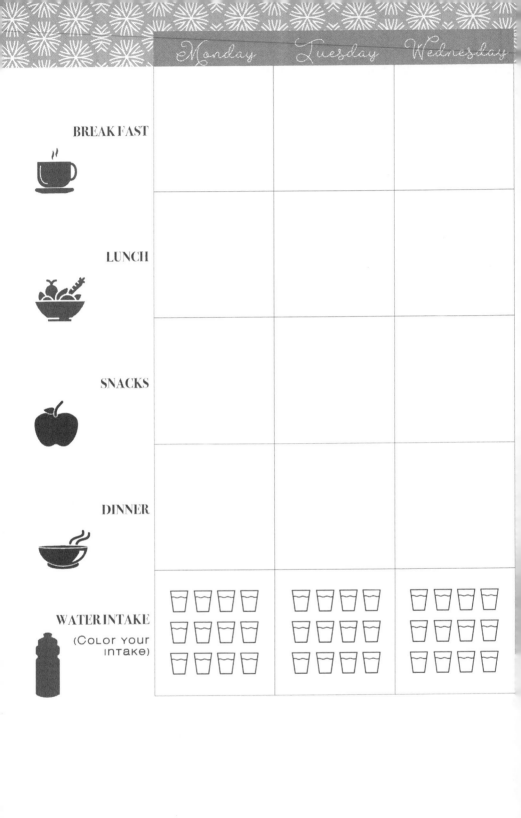

	Monday	Tuesday	Wednesday
BREAKFAST			
LUNCH			
SNACKS			
DINNER			
WATER INTAKE (Color your intake)			

Thursday	Friday	Saturday	Sunday

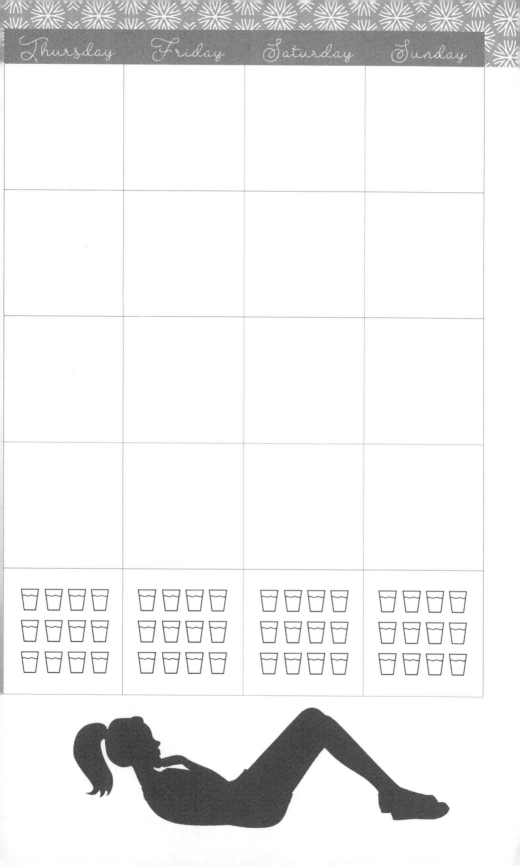

Plan
AHEAD

Date: _____ _____ TO _____ _____

	Current	Goal
Weight:		
Body fat %:		
Energy Level:		
Other:		

This week's plan

Work out schedule: **S M T W T F S**

Nutrition: _____

_____

_____

Goals: _____

_____

_____

Reward

_____

_____

_____

_____

_____

Notes

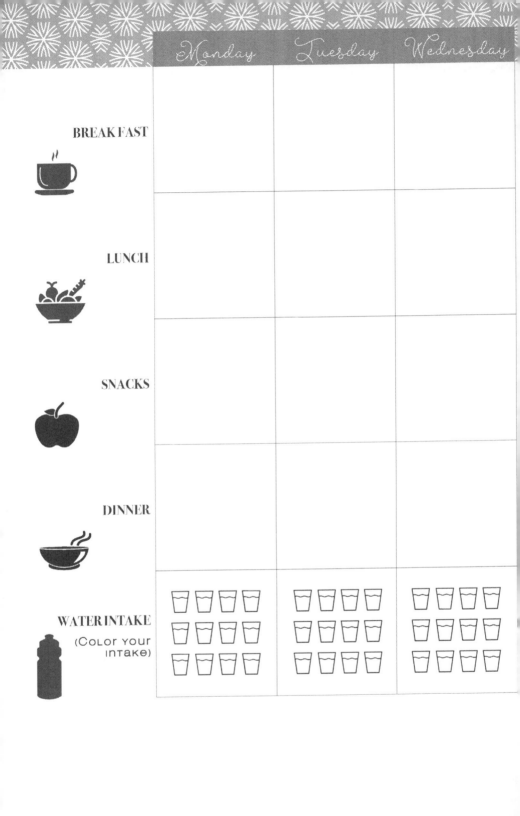

	Monday	Tuesday	Wednesday
BREAKFAST			
LUNCH			
SNACKS			
DINNER			
WATER INTAKE (Color your intake)			

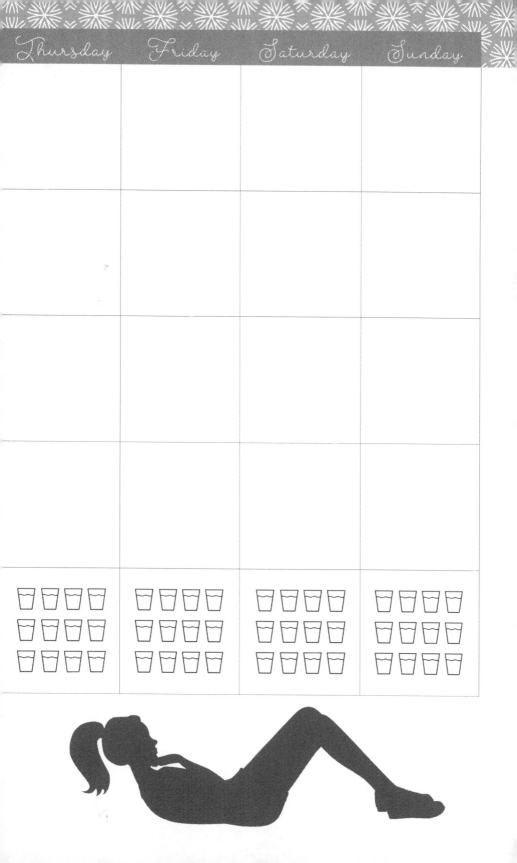

Plan
AHEAD

Date: _____ _____ _____ TO _____ _____ _____

	Current	Goal
Weight:		
Body fat %:		
Energy level:		
Other:		

This week's plan

Work out schedule: **S   M   T   W   T   F   S**

Nutrition: _____

_____

_____

Goals: _____

_____

_____

Reward

_____

_____

_____

_____

_____

Notes

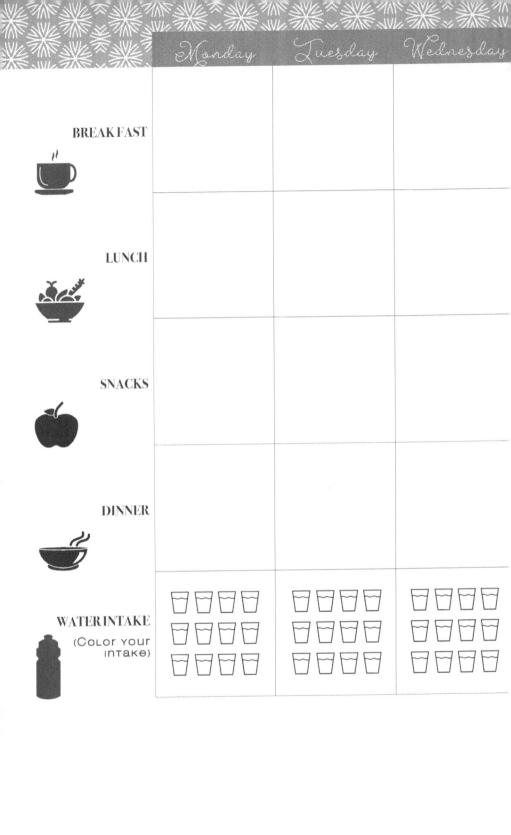

	Monday	Tuesday	Wednesday
BREAKFAST			
LUNCH			
SNACKS			
DINNER			
WATER INTAKE (Color your intake)			

Thursday	Friday	Saturday	Sunday

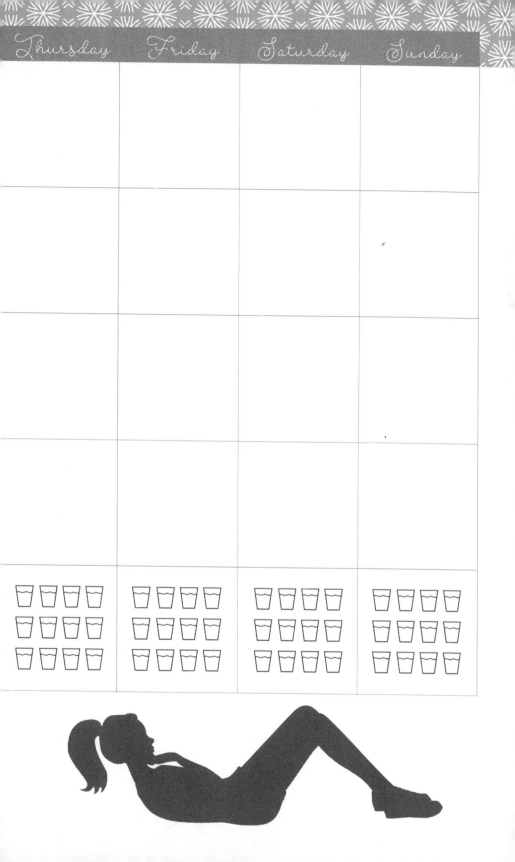

Plan
AHEAD

Date: _____ _____ _____ TO _____ _____ _____

	Current	Goal
WEIGHT:		
BODY FAT %:		
ENERGY LEVEL:		
OTHER:		

This week's plan

WORK OUT SCHEDULE: **S M T W T F S**

NUTRITION: _____
_____
_____

GOALS: _____
_____
_____

Reward

_____
_____
_____
_____

Notes

	Monday	Tuesday	Wednesday
BREAKFAST 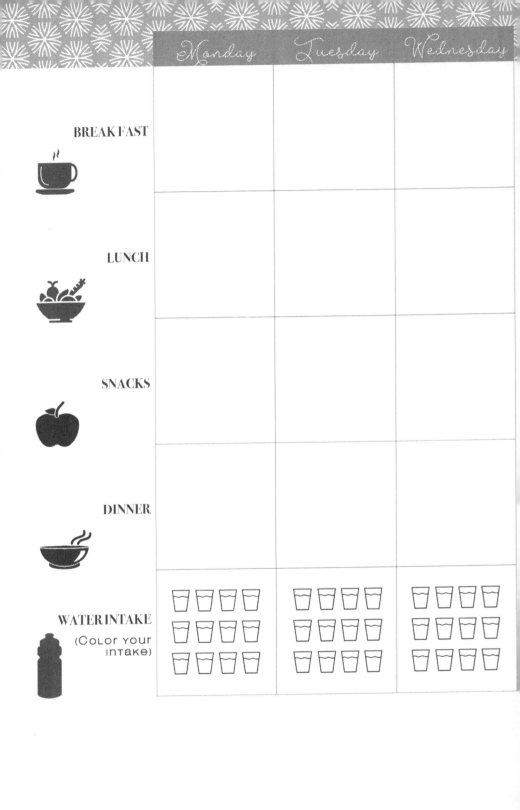			
LUNCH			
SNACKS			
DINNER			
WATER INTAKE (Color your intake)			

Thursday	Friday	Saturday	Sunday

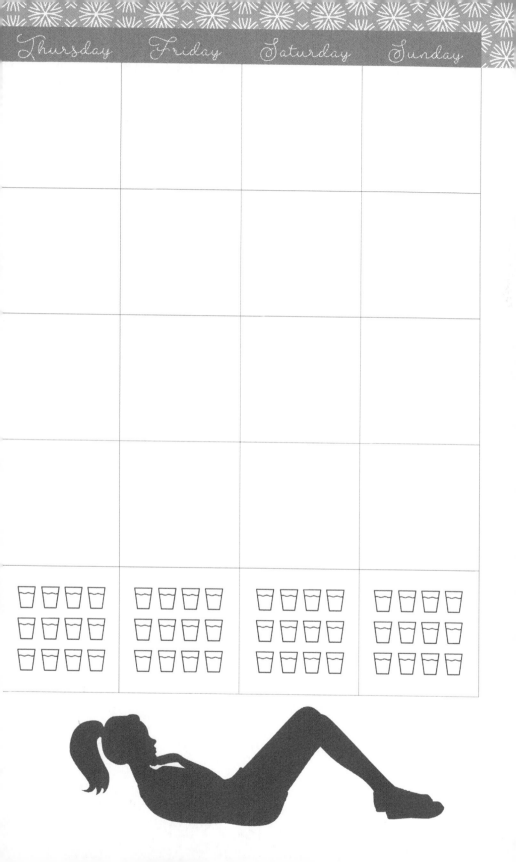

Work OUTS

Strength Training

Exercise	Reps.	Sets	Focus

Notes

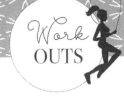

Work OUTS

CARDIO: Exercise   Duration   Cals. Burned

_____   _____   _____
_____   _____   _____
_____   _____   _____

STRETCH: Cool-down   TIME

_____   _____
_____   _____
_____   _____

Workout TRACKER

1	2	3	4	5	6	7	8
9	10	11	12	13	14	15	16
17	18	19	20	21	22	23	24
25	26	27	28	29	30	31	

Habits TRACKER

Everyday habits

1 _____   4 _____
2 _____   5 _____
3 _____   6 _____

	1	2	3	4	5	6		1	2	3	4	5	6
1							17						
2							18						
3							19						
4							20						
5							21						
6							22						
7							23						
8							24						
9							25						
10							26						
11							27						
12							28						
13							29						
14							30						
15							31						
16													

Plan
AHEAD

Date: _____ _____ TO _____ _____

	Current	Goal
Weight:		
Body fat %:		
Energy Level:		
Other:		

This week's plan

Work out schedule: S   M   T   W   T   F   S

Nutrition: _____
_____
_____

Goals: _____
_____
_____

Reward

_____
_____
_____
_____
_____

Notes

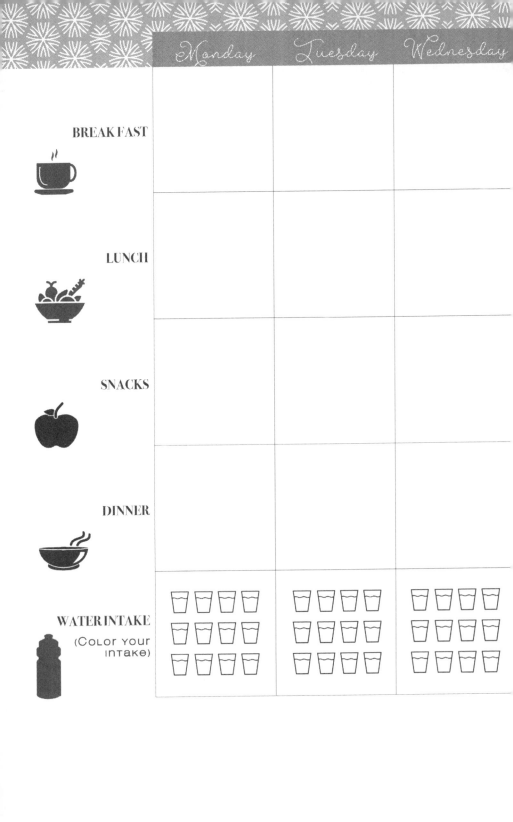

	Monday	Tuesday	Wednesday
BREAKFAST			
LUNCH			
SNACKS			
DINNER			
WATER INTAKE (Color your intake)			

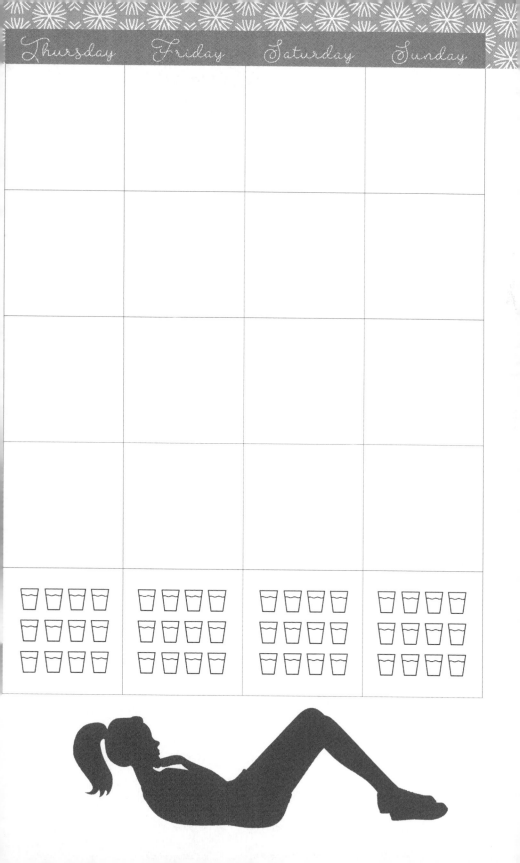

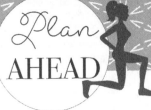

Plan AHEAD

Date: _____ _____ _____   TO _____ _____ _____

	Current	Goal
Weight:		
Body fat %:		
Energy Level:		
Other:		

This week's plan

Work out schedule: **S   M   T   W   T   F   S**

Nutrition: _____
_____
_____

Goals: _____
_____
_____

Reward

_____
_____
_____
_____
_____

Notes

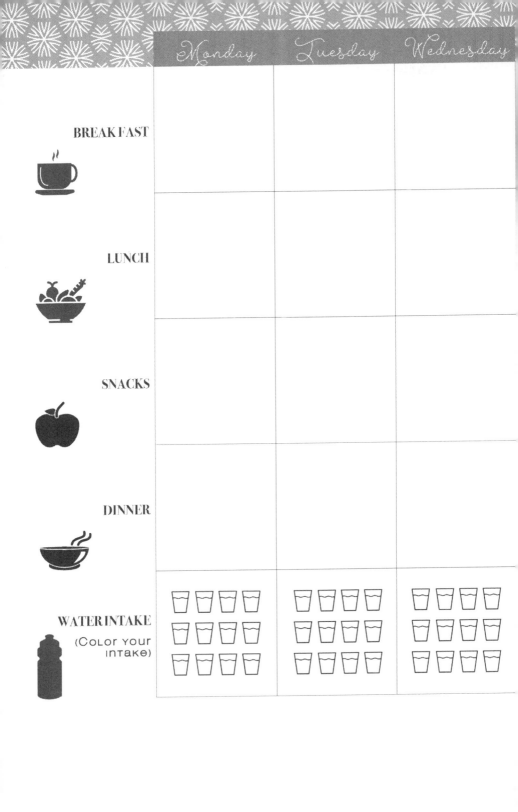

	Monday	Tuesday	Wednesday
BREAKFAST			
LUNCH			
SNACKS			
DINNER			
WATER INTAKE (Color your intake)			

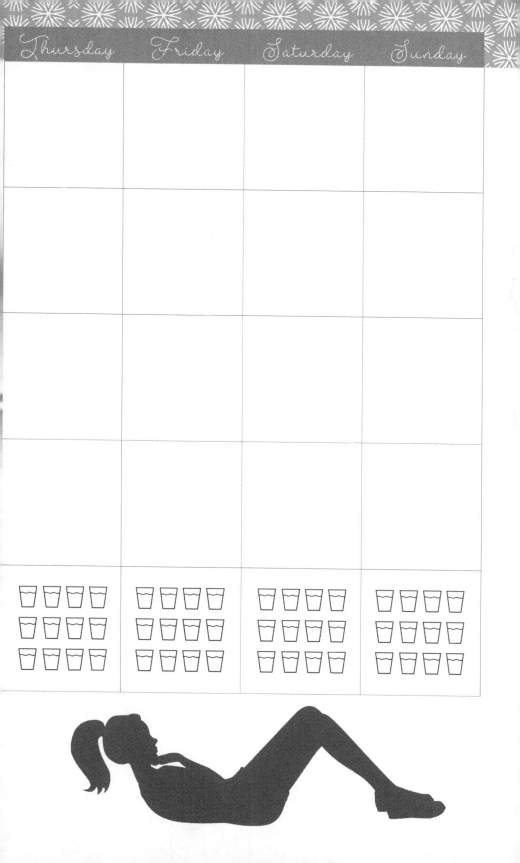

Plan
AHEAD

Date: _____ TO _____

	Current	Goal
Weight:		
Body fat %:		
Energy Level:		
Other:		

This week's plan

Work out schedule: S M T W T F S

Nutrition: _____

_____

_____

Goals: _____

_____

_____

Reward

_____

_____

_____

_____

Notes

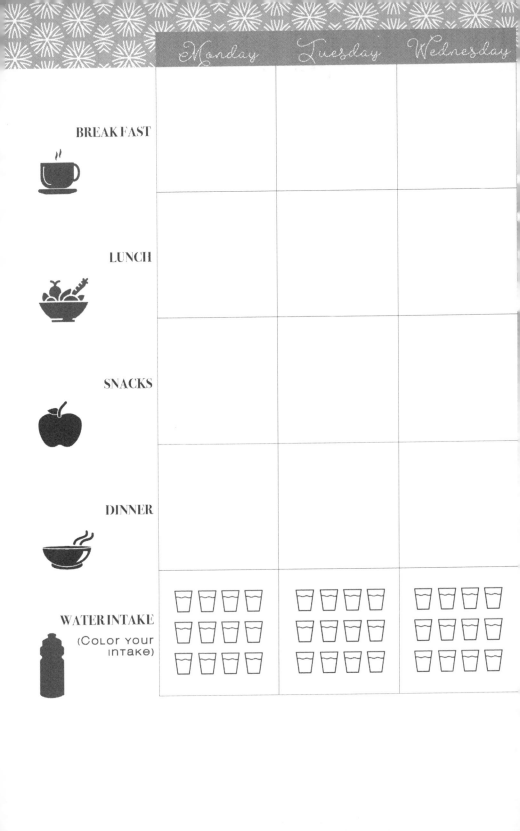

	Monday	Tuesday	Wednesday
BREAKFAST			
LUNCH			
SNACKS			
DINNER			
WATER INTAKE (Color your intake)			

| --- | --- | --- | --- |

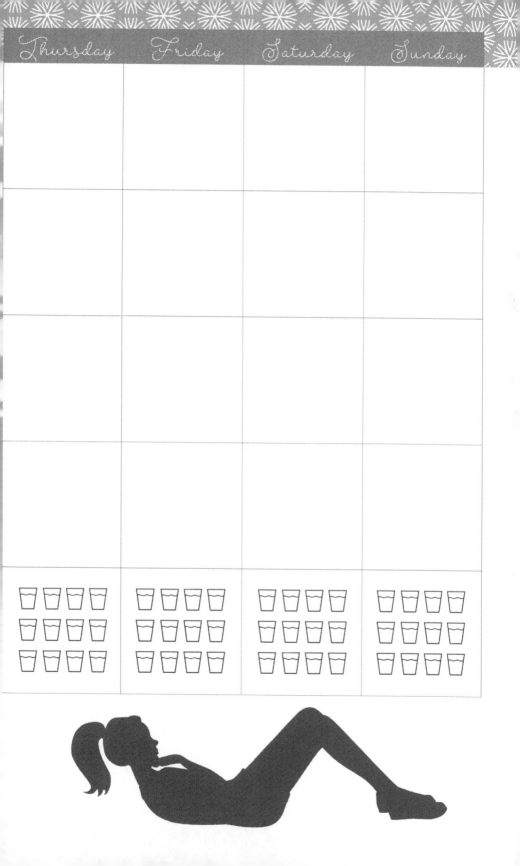

Plan
AHEAD

Date: _____ _____ _____   TO _____ _____ _____

	Current	Goal
Weight:		
Body fat %:		
Energy Level:		
Other:		

This week's plan

Work out schedule: S   M   T   W   T   F   S

Nutrition: _____
_____
_____

Goals: _____
_____
_____

Reward

_____
_____
_____
_____
_____

Notes

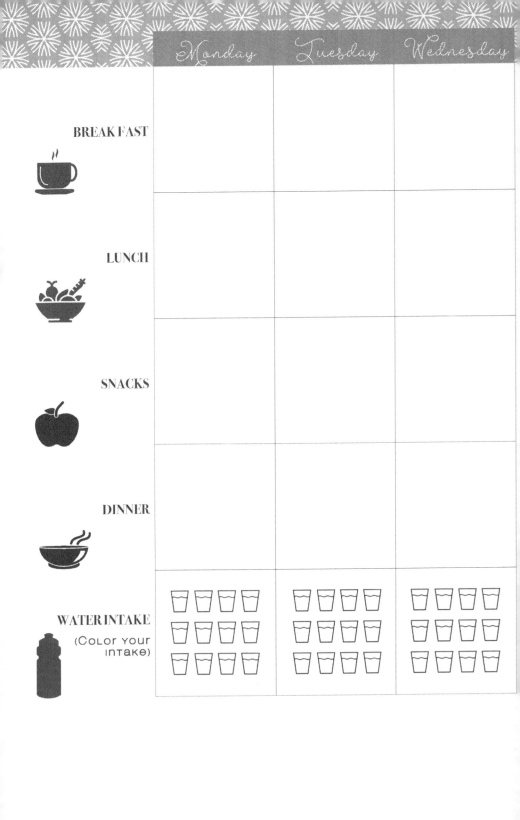

	Monday	Tuesday	Wednesday
BREAKFAST			
LUNCH			
SNACKS			
DINNER			
WATER INTAKE (Color your intake)			

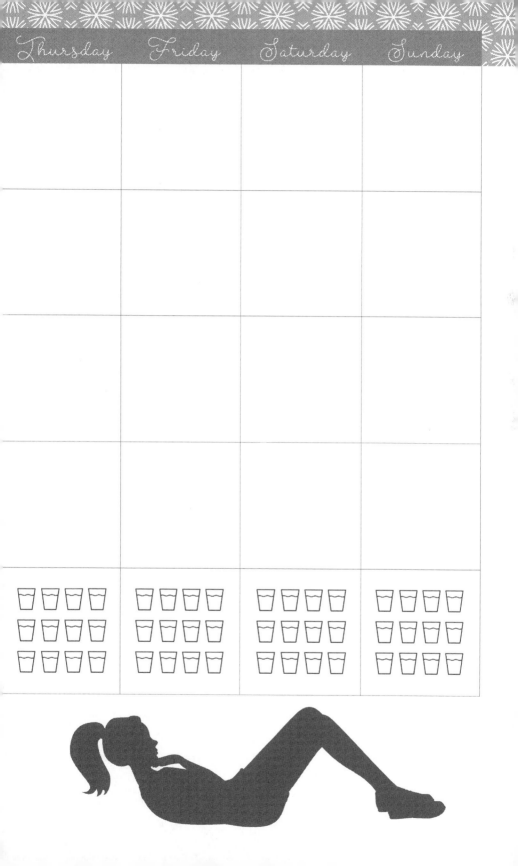

Strength Training

Exercise	Reps.	Sets	Focus

Notes

65389352R00150

Made in the USA
Middletown, DE
02 September 2019